A CAREGIVER'S GUIDE TO DEMENTIA

What If It's Not
ALZHEIMER'S?

A CAREGIVER'S GUIDE TO DEMENTIA

What If It's Not
ALZHEIMER'S?

Includes Vital Information on
FRONTOTEMPORAL DEMENTIA (FTD)

edited by
Lisa Radin & Gary Radin

foreword by Murray Grossman, M.D., Ed.D.

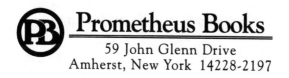 Prometheus Books

59 John Glenn Drive
Amherst, New York 14228-2197

Published 2003 by Prometheus Books

What If It's Not Alzheimer's? Copyright © 2003 by Lisa Radin and Gary Radin. All rights reserved. No part of this publication may be reproduced, stored in a retrieval system, or transmitted in any form or by any means, digital, electronic, mechanical, photocopying, recording, or otherwise, or conveyed via the Internet or a Web site without prior written permission of the publisher, except in the case of brief quotations embodied in critical articles and reviews.

Inquiries should be addressed to
Prometheus Books
59 John Glenn Drive
Amherst, New York 14228–2197
VOICE: 716–691–0133, ext. 207
FAX: 716–564–2711

07 06 05   5 4 3

Library of Congress Cataloging-in-Publication Data

What if it's not Alzheimer's : a caregiver's guide to dementia / edited by Lisa
    Radin and Gary Radin.
        p. cm.
    Includes bibliographical references and index.
    ISBN 1–59102–087–5 (pbk. alk. paper)
        1. Dementia—Nursing—Handbooks, manuals, etc. 2. Dementia—Patients—
Care—Handbooks, manuals, etc. 3. Caregivers—Handbooks, manuals, etc.
[DNLM: 1. Dementia—diagnosis—Handbooks. 2. Dementia—nursing—Hand-
books. 3. Activities of Daily Living—Handbooks. 4. Caregivers—psychology—
Handbooks. 5. Family Relations—Handbooks. 6. Home Nursing—methods—
Handbooks. WM 34 W555 2003] I. Radin, Lisa, 1944– II. Radin, Gary, 1969–

RC521.W438 2003
616.8'3—dc21

                                                                2003010851

Printed in the United States on acid-free paper

*This book is dedicated to
our loving husband and father, Neil, and
to all those who walk in our footsteps
through the journey of FTD.*

Contents

PART IV: Caring for Yourself

Foreword

believe that an important function of a physician is to educate the patient and the patient's family. This becomes increasingly difficult as physicians are forced to spend less meaningful time in conversation with patients. *What If It's Not Alzheimer's? A Caregiver's Guide to Dementia* serves a crucial role in the medical care of patients with frontotemporal dementia since much of the educational function of physicians is represented in its pages.

The broad-based content of this volume addresses both the medical elements of frontotemporal dementia that are important for patients and families to understand, and many of the practical issues relating to care on a day-to-day basis. This is particularly important for families and caregivers of patients with frontotemporal dementia, since this condition interrupts critical social and communicative functions that we often take for granted.

In many ways, this book also is a model for opening communication with families of patients suffering from slowly progressive neurologic conditions, and I hope that practitioners in other areas will view this volume as a challenge to develop similar programs in other areas of medicine and neurology.

Murray Grossman, M.D., Ed.D.
Department of Neurology
University of Pennsylvania Medical Center

Preface

The publication of this caregiver manual is very exciting! There has been a great need for a book combining accurate information about frontotemporal dementia with practical information for caregivers. *What If It's Not Alzheimer's? A Caregiver's Guide to Dementia* meets this need.

My husband, Craig, was diagnosed with Pick's disease in 1979. That was a time when very few people had heard about Alzheimer's disease, and almost no one had heard about Pick's disease or frontotemporal dementia. There were no brochures. There were very few published papers. There was no book to consult. As I cared for my husband, I often felt as if I were laying railroad tracks and trying very hard to finish ahead of the train that was bearing down on me. Sometimes the train overtook me.

After my husband died, I became executive director of the Southeastern Pennsylvania chapter of the Alzheimer's Association. During my fifteen-year tenure, I saw an increasing number of people contacting the chapter for information and tips on caring for someone with frontotemporal dementia. There was little information for us to give them. It would have been so helpful to have a caregiver manual to guide the way.

It is for all these reasons that the publication of this book gives me great pleasure. I am happy to recommend the manual to those who are coping with frontotemporal dementia. It will be an *invaluable* resource!

Helen-Ann Comstock
Caregiver for husband, 1978–1984
Chair, The Association for Frontotemporal Dementias

Acknowledgments

Creating a book of this scope was no small task. However, in light of the monumental difference it could make in the lives of those caring for someone with frontotemporal dementia, it was worth every minute. The idea of assembling the thoughts, knowledge, and expertise of this ensemble of talented professionals and caregivers was both exciting and overwhelming. The number of titles and credentials following the names of the writers in this book is impressive. They are experts who have dedicated their lives to caring and providing for people whose loved ones have FTD, as well as researching and contributing to the future care of FTD patients.

We also owe our gratitude to the many families, friends, and professionals, too numerous to mention, that supported us and cared for our loved one during the most difficult time of our life. You are truly at the source of our commitment to take our experience and turn it into something that will help others as they face the role of caregiving.

We are so grateful and thankful for the incredible generosity that each and every contributor has made to this endeavor. Their efforts go far beyond the writing of this book. They offer information, guidance, and hope for all those who come into contact with the challenges and reality of living with FTD.

We want to thank Murray Grossman, M.D., Ed.D., for the ongoing encouragement to create this book and for his personal commitment to patients and families dealing with dementia. He is a role model for the medical profession. Jennifer Farmer, M.S., C.G.C., has given spirit, knowledge, and many hours to ensure that we have included everything caregivers need to know and that all the contributors to this book have been well represented. She is an angel that descended upon this project. Helen-Ann Comstock is a pioneer in supporting, educating, advocating, and loving both caregivers and FTD patients in need in our region. Carol Lippa, M.D., has proven time and again that caregivers and their loved ones deserve knowledge they can understand and take home into everyday life. We also acknowledge the contributing authors, without whom this book would never have been possible: Jeannette Castellane, L.S.W.; Tiffany W. Chow, M.D.; Heather J. Cianci, P.T., G.C.S.; Helen-Ann Comstock; Rev. David Cotton; Lisa Ann Fagan, O.T.R./L., C.A.L.A.; Jennifer Farmer, M.S., C.G.C.; Paul L. Feldman, Esq.; Judy L. Fisher, R.N., M.S., Ph.D. candidate; Rosalie Gearhart, R.N., M.S., C.S.; Jordan Grafman, Ph.D.; Vivian Greenberg, A.C.S.W., L.C.S.W.; Murray Grossman, M.D., Ed.D.; Kent S. Jamison, Ph.D.; Morris Kaplan, Esq., N.H.A.; Virginia M.-Y. Lee, Ph.D.; Carol F. Lippa, M.D.; Bruce L. Miller, M.D.; Kate Rankin, Ph.D.; Susan Riley, L.S.W.; Keith M. Robinson, M.D.; Martin Rosser, M.A., M.D., F.R.C.P.; John Q. Trojanowski, M.D., Ph.D.; Erica Wollman, M.Ed., C.C.C.-S.L.P.

In addition, we'd like to thank the Alzheimer's Association Delaware Valley Chapter, Pick's Support Group for its love, caregiver words of wisdom, and bravery in the face of fear; Fytie Drayton and Joyce Shenian, special caregivers and friends, who have given their blessing for this book and invaluable feedback and unconditional support to all those around them; all the caregivers who responded to our questionnaire; our close family and friends for their interest and support—especially Geri for her love and compassion and Vince for his ongoing patience, humor, and willingness to let us disappear as we worked for hours and even days at a time.

Introduction

I t is years since our bodies have recovered from the incredibly challenging task of caring for a loved one, yet our minds still have vivid memories of the overwhelming experience. We are the wife and son of an intelligent, loving, and generous husband and father. We are the caregivers of a beautiful man who died at age fifty-eight after suffering from a neurodegenerative dementia.

Our four years of providing in-home care unraveled a series of events that we discovered no one could ever be prepared for. Every day included the challenges of what doctors to consult, where to go for financial assistance, who could provide us with support, how to get information and when we would ever deal with the loss. We were driven to find answers to questions that would help us understand, cope, and manage and put us on a path to learn everything we could from every source we could find. Finding almost nothing, the only answer we did see to make it through was to pave our own road.

What If It's Not Alzheimer's? A Caregiver's Guide to Dementia is a map of the road we traveled. It is a collection of information addressing everything we had to confront and conquer while caring for our loved one. Medical professionals and experienced caregivers, many of whom are renowned for their work, write the pages of these chapters. Some are the same people we personally sought out and from whom we asked advice. Providing the information that every caregiver seeks, this volume encompasses all the facts that would take monumental efforts to gather together.

Giant steps are being taken in this book to direct focus on the group of brain disorders known collectively as frontotemporal dementia (FTD). This classification of progressive, neurodegenerative dementias, along with many other non-Alzheimer's diseases, have been overshadowed or even eclipsed by the dominance of funded research and awareness campaigns for Alzheimer's disease. Although concentration on Alzheimer's disease over the past twenty years has provided significant medical developments and needed public attention, it is critical that we now take a step back and acknowledge the *many* different degenerative conditions that affect the brain.

The medical profession has been distinguishing dementia illnesses in greater depth in the past few years. As a result, diagnosis has led to other dementias as clinical observations rule out Alzheimer's. For this reason, the medical community and our ever-growing caregiving society must educate itself and disseminate the distinctions that will provide better treatment and care to those afflicted with FTD and related disorders.

Non-Alzheimer's disorders are often considered rare; however, they are not actually that uncommon. It could be said that FTD is often misdiagnosed and underrecognized. This is also true of the numerous other non-Alzheimer's disorders, which present both subtle and not so subtle differences from Alzheimer's disease. This guidebook presents both caregiver advice and information along with medical discussion and experience specifically targeted at FTD but absolutely relevant to other dementias. We also think it is equally useful and informative to the healthcare community by presenting insight into caregiver daily needs as well as a comprehensive perspective on medical care.

Too many people struggle with unanswered questions, little direction, and no diagnosis, sometimes for as long as years. Others are misdiagnosed with personality and psychological conditions only to later find out there is a neurodegenerative condition that is the cause of the matter. For this reason, the information that follows will be useful to caregivers who are moving down the road and to professionals who are directing them.

For you, the caregiver, we understand what lies ahead. It is a difficult time and certainly an emotional one. Your commitment to provide the best quality of life for your loved one is recognized. And we know that the time and energy it takes is unparalleled. Be strong, fearless, and, most of all, keep on loving the one you care for as well as yourself.

This book is part of our mission to take our experience and make a difference in the lives of those who are now suffering with FTD. Read these pages one by one. Use each chapter in every way you can to provide the knowledge and power that will sustain you in your time of caregiving.

Editors' Note

This guidebook is written with the intention of providing accurate and timely information. The subject matter has been addressed with care and concern for caregivers and respect for healthcare and other professionals. There is a great amount of detail from numerous sources and we have attempted to organize it in a manner that allows you to reference relevant information at any time.

We acknowledge that there are many different types of relationships involved in caregiving, but for the purposes of literary clarity we may not have been able to mention all people in the text. Those afflicted with neurodegenerative illnesses and their caregivers are both men and women. To simplify reading we use only one pronoun (i.e., he or she) at a time and switch continually throughout the book.

Information at the time of publishing can be considered correct and current; however, due to ongoing research, new practices, changes in law, etc., additional information and facts will arise over time and may change. This book is for informational purposes only and is not intended to provide medical or legal advice. Health conditions and treatments are unique to every individual, and medical or other professionals should be consulted for each individual circumstance.

Part I
A Medical Focus

CHAPTER I

The ABCs of Neurodegenerative Dementias

MARTIN ROSSOR

WHAT IS DEMENTIA?

The most common cause of dementia is Alzheimer's disease (AD), which has dominated our thinking about neurodegenerative disorders and even determined the definition of the term "dementia" itself. It is clear, however, that there are many other causes of dementia. Before discussing these it is first necessary to consider what is meant by dementia and the history behind it.

The term "dementia" refers to a clinical syndrome, a combination or pattern of clinical features. Thus, dementia is not a disease, but rather a syndrome that can be associated with many different underlying diseases. In this sense it is similar to heartburn or headache, which is caused by many different things and could require many different treatments. Therefore, the statement that somebody has dementia is an inadequate diagnostic formulation: One must always try to determine the cause by appropriate investigations.

With the syndrome dementia, impairment of cognitive function is widespread. It can involve, in different combinations, memory for events; memory and understanding of facts, language, thinking, and reasoning; and perception of the world. Identifying patients with this combination of cognitive impairment was particularly important in the days before imaging (e.g., MRI and CT). It was important to distinguish patients with a localized deficit from those with more widespread problems. Cognitive function in the brain is modular and particular areas of the cerebral cortex are specialized for particular functions; for example, our ability to remember day-to-day events is critically dependant upon the hippocampus, found on the inside of the temporal lobes. (see figure 1.)

THE BRAIN

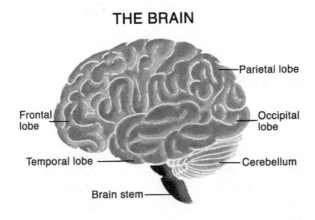

Figure 1: Illustration of the major areas of the brain.

What the Different Parts of the Brain Do

Cerebrum: This is the term for the entire cerebral cortex (outside of the brain). The cerebrum is responsible for many aspects of thinking, including memory, problem solving, language function, personality, mood, and response to different sensory signals from the world around us. It also plays a role in movement and in feeling the senses. It is highly developed in humans, but more rudimentary in animals.

Cerebellum: Coordinates, smoothes out, and balances movement to enable individuals to stand, walk, and use their arms.

Frontal lobe: This part of the brain controls our ability to use words and speech (the left side) and determines how we react to situations emotionally. The frontal lobes are also important for energy, problem solving, mood, judgment, inhibiting impulses, and for individual personality.

Parietal lobe: This part of the brain enables one to interpret sensory input such as pain, temperature differences, vibration, and touch. The right parietal lobe is also important for our sense of direction.

Occipital lobe: This part of the brain interprets what one sees.

Temporal lobes: The temporal lobes are crucial for formation of new memories (remembering). This part of the brain is always involved in Alzheimer's disease and may be involved in frontotemporal dementia. The left temporal lobe is also important for understanding what we hear.

Brain stem: Connects the brain with the spinal cord. Without the brainstem we wouldn't be able to move or feel anything. This area is also important for automatic reflexes such as breathing.

By contrast, our language functions are critically dependant on areas of the left frontal and temporal cortex in right-handed people. Patients with a discrete abnormality, such as a loss of language or dysphasia, by implication would have a focal or localized damage to the cerebral cortex. If this were of sudden onset it would likely be a stroke, but if it were of slow onset then it would likely be a tumor and thus require invasive and potentially dangerous investigation and surgery. On the other hand, a patient with widespread deficits would likely have a disease more diffusely affecting the cerebral cortex, such as Alzheimer's disease, and further investigation could be avoided. Historically the terms "senile" and "presenile dementia" were used merely to refer to dementias coming on late or early in life. These were most likely to be Alzheimer's disease, but again this was not a specific diagnosis as such.

More recently the definition of dementia has been made more precise. The necessity for more than one cognitive domain to be involved remains critical to the definition; however, memory, and particularly our ability to remember day-to-day events (episodic memory), has to be affected for dementia to occur. Alzheimer's disease, in which episodic memory is the most salient deficit, is the most common dementia disorder. In addition to memory impairment, there has to be at least one other domain of cognitive impairment such as language, thinking, or perception. Furthermore, the cognitive impairment has to be significant enough to interfere with social or employment functions. In other words, the patient must be quite severely affected.

The different degenerative diseases that can cause the dementia syndrome tend to affect different areas of the cerebral cortex. Since different areas of the cortex are specialized for different functions, the disease will tend to have characteristic patterns of deficit. This is most apparent early in the disease. As the disease progresses they tend to become more similar as dysfunction becomes more severe and more widespread. Clearly, as we move toward earlier diagnosis, essential to successful management of these diseases in the future, we will attempt to diagnose them before a patient fulfills the criteria for dementia. For example, a patient with early Alzheimer's disease may present with mild memory deficit, but this alone is not sufficient to fulfill the criteria for dementia. Similarly, many patients with a frontotemporal dementia may have preserved memory early in the disease but demonstrate quite profound behavioral and personality changes. For these reasons, many specialists now believe we should begin to move away from the term "dementia" and to speak in terms of specific patterns of cognitive impairment and the relationship to presumed underlying diseases.

FRONTOTEMPORAL DEMENTIA

The frontotemporal dementias (FTD) comprise the main topic of this book, and the clinical and pathological details are discussed in the following chapters. However, the key feature of this group of disorders is the involvement of a variety of disease processes of the frontal lobes and the front part of the temporal lobes of the brain. It is this characteristic distribution or topography of the degenerative process that determines the clinical features of early personality change, language, and speech impairment. There are many different underlying diseases that can present as a frontotemporal dementia. Some of these are quite specific, such as Pick's disease. Pick's disease was identified even earlier than Alzheimer's disease. Arnold Pick in Prague described two patients with prominent behavioral and language impairment. Intriguingly it was Alzheimer who again applied his expertise with the microscope to the examination of the brain and demonstrated some abnormal inclusions subsequently referred to as Pick bodies. These are now known to be deposits of tau protein. The tau protein that is deposited in Pick's disease is the same as that found in the neurofibrillary tangles of Alzheimer's disease, but is deposited in a different way. Senile plaques are not a feature of Pick's disease.

The term "Pick's disease" has been somewhat confusing, since it has been used both as a general clinical term, essentially the same as frontotemporal dementia, as well as a very specific pathological disease. Increasingly it is used in the latter sense.

Corticobasal degeneration (CBD) is another disease of abnormal tau. Typically it affects the parietal lobe and causes major difficulty with motor skills but can affect the frontal and temporal lobes, causing FTD.

Some cases of FTD show abnormalities under the microscope that are similar to those found in another degenerative disorder, motor neuron disease or Lou Gehrig's disease, also known as ALS. Other patients may show no specific features when the brain is examined under the microscope and it is probable that this is a very heterogeneous group that we will gradually understand better over time.

It is the early behavioral and personality changes and/or changes in language and speech that define this group of patients. Their memory for day-to-day events may be strikingly preserved when compared with Alzheimer's disease, and they very rarely if ever get lost until late in the disease. Three prototypic clinical syndromes have been described in association with FTD: a frontal dysexecutive syndrome, progressive nonfluent aphasia, and semantic dementia. The frontal syndrome is characterized by behavioral abnormalities. Patients become socially disinhibited, with some becoming aggressive and others apathetic. There may be changes in eating and sexual behavior. The term "frontotemporal dementia" is sometimes confined to this group. Progressive nonfluent aphasia refers to patients with speech production difficulties. Early on, they have excellent comprehension and may write well despite speaking with difficulty. As the disease progresses they become mute. Semantic dementia refers to patients with impairment of semantic memory. This term refers to our knowledge of meaning. Verbal semantic memory is our memory for the meaning of words and visual semantic memory is our memory for the meaning of objects that we see. Semantic memory contrasts with our memory for day-to-day events, referred to as episodic memory. Patients with semantic memory speak fluently but it is empty of meaning and they have major difficulty understanding. With this condition there is loss of tissue in the temporal lobes.

DEMENTIA WITH LEWY BODIES

Dementia with Lewy bodies (DLB) has been increasingly identified as an important cause of dementia in the elderly. In some studies it is believed to be the cause of dementia in up to 20 percent of the patients in this age group. Under the microscope, the brains of people with DLB show the senile plaques of Alzheimer's disease but far fewer neurofibrillary tangles. By contrast, they show the brain cell changes that are normally associated with Parkinson's disease, that is, a protein deposit referred to as a Lewy body, named after its original discoverer.

Patients with DLB more closely resemble patients with Alzheimer's disease than those with FTD. There is a characteristic clinical triad that favors the diagnosis, namely fluctuation in the cognitive impairment, hallucinations, and Parkinsonian syndrome.

The fluctuations in cognitive impairment can be quite dramatic and last from minutes to days. In between times the family will often feel that the patient is normal, at least early in the disease. The hallucinations are very frequent and patients rapidly regain insight. They are normally of people and animals. The people may often be familiar to them and distressingly may be deceased relatives or friends. The hallucinations are rarely threatening and rarely speak to the patients. They commonly accompany misidentifications of objects in their environments. For example, an abnormally hanging curtain may be seen as a figure that then takes the form of a more definite hallucination.

The Parkinsonian syndrome is very similar to that seen in patients with classical Parkinson's disease. There is a gradual slowing of movement and of rigidity, but the tremor or shakiness of classical Parkinson's disease is less often seen.

ALZHEIMER'S DISEASE

It is often claimed that there is an epidemic of Alzheimer's disease. The disease has always been with us, but since it is a disease of old age, the numbers of cases have increased with the aging of the population. The real increase, however, has been due to current diagnosis, whereas thirty years ago many patients would simply have been diagnosed as suffering from senile dementia.

Alzheimer's original case was a lady of only fifty-one years of age who presented with dementia. Alzheimer examined her brain after death using the newly available silver stains. He was thus able to demonstrate the two characteristic microscopic features: senile plaques and neurofibrillary tangles. Senile plaques are now known to reflect deposits of an abnormal protein, beta-amyloid, within the brain but not within the neurons or brain cells themselves; this is thought to be a key event in the causation of the disease. Neurofibrillary tangles are now known to be abnormal deposits of another protein within the cell itself. This protein is tau, the microtubule-associated protein. Microtubules are the building blocks of the internal skeleton of brain cells and essential to maintain the integrity of the extensive and complex wiring within the brain. If tau loses its function then microtubules become unstable, and one can see the collapse of the cytoskeleton as neurofibrillary tangles.

Since Alzheimer's first case was a middle-aged lady it was assumed that this was a rare early onset or presenile dementia. However, studies in the United Kingdom in the 1960s demonstrated that the majority of elderly patients with dementia, which had previously been called senile dementia, were in fact suffering from Alzheimer's disease.

The key clinical feature of Alzheimer's disease is an early impairment of episodic memory, our memory for day-to-day events. Patients may have difficulty recalling what has happened to them; they forget to do things; they may misplace items; they repetitively question; and as the disease progresses, they may get lost. We all experience these features from time to time but it is the inexorable progression that identifies the patient with early Alzheimer's disease. After a period of a few years, other features supervene with increasing difficulties with language and perception of the world. This pattern reflects the early involvement of the hippocampus, as explained previously, and other parts of the temporal lobe by the disease process.

VASCULAR DEMENTIA

It used to be thought that impairment of blood supply to the brain was the main cause of dementia. It was believed that hardening of the arteries, or atherosclerosis, led to a reduced blood flow. This has been disproved. While blood flow may be reduced in dementia, this is a consequence of the nerve cell loss rather than a cause. What can cause dementia is recurrent large or small strokes and nerve cell damage from disease in the small arteries to the central parts of the brain, called small vessel disease or Binswanger's disease.

Patients with strokes can have significant problems with cognitive impairment, such as a patient with a right-sided paralysis accompanying loss of language or dysphasia. Multiple strokes can give rise to widespread cognitive impairment, but due to motor abnormalities, it is usually obvious that these are strokes and such patients rarely come to attention because of the cognitive impairment alone. Occasionally, a stroke in particular areas of the cerebral cortex or in the center of the brain (in the thalamus), can result in quite widespread cognitive impairment.

Much more common are the consequences of high blood pressure, smoking, and diabetes in patients with dementia. These conspire to cause thickening and damage to the very small arteries that supply the center of the brain with oxygen and result in little ministrokes or lacunas together with more diffuse damage to the central white matter of the brain. These patients often present with cognitive impairment or dementia. They tend to be characterized by cognitive slowing and often have problems with recall but not with recognition memory. Gait disturbance, which can resemble Parkinson's disease with shuffling, is quite common. This is an important group of patients to identify. Careful management of risk factors such as blood pressure, cholesterol, and blood sugar are important and may slow progress. In addition, many patients with Alzheimer's disease have coincidental vascular disease and it is believed that the vascular disease may exacerbate the Alzheimer pathology changes.

OTHER DEGENERATIVE DISEASES

Alzheimer's disease, frontotemporal dementia, and dementia with Lewy bodies are the three main groups of degenerative diseases causing dementia, that is, diseases with direct and progressive loss of brain cells. There are other degenerative diseases that can cause dementia, such as Huntington's disease and progressive supranuclear palsy or Steele Richardson syndrome, but with these there are often other neurological abnormalities such as problems with walking. Creutzfeldt-Jakob disease (CJD) is a very distressing and rapidly progressive degenerative disorder that can lead to death in a matter of months. In Europe, cases of variant CJD are now being seen which are believed to be linked to bovine spongiform encephalopathy or mad cow disease. In all of the degenerative dementias the underlying disease process tends to affect particular areas of the brain or particular groups of cells. It is this selective vulnerability that determines the early clinical features. These are very important diagnostic clues for the neurologist and psychiatrist.

OTHER CAUSES OF DEMENTIA

The causes of dementia and/or less severe cognitive impairment are innumerable. Many of the causes give rise to cognitive slowing or mild cognitive impairment rather than the panoply of severe dementia. However, as patients are presenting earlier, it is important to undertake very careful investigation and consideration of the full differential diagnosis. Patients with a frontal meningioma, a benign tumor, can still present late with slowly progressive personality change and emerging dementia. Chronic infections such as tuberculous meningitis can also give rise to cognitive impairment, as can HIV disease.

Drug-induced dementia is an important group to consider. The elderly in particular can be quite sensitive to side effects of many medications. Sleeping tablets are notorious for causing memory lapses. Alcohol also can cause cognitive impairment and the history is not always obvious. In some patients with poor nutrition and very high alcohol intake, Korsakov's syndrome occurs with a very severe memory deficit. Depression is another important cause to consider. Many patients with depression will complain of their memory and can be shown to have a genuine cognitive slowing. In severe, untreated depression this can resemble Alzheimer's disease. The clinical situation is complicated by the fact that depression is common in early Alzheimer's disease. Therefore, even if there is improvement in cognition following a trial of an antidepressant, the patient may still go on to progress to a clinically definite Alzheimer's disease. If in doubt, such a patient should always have a trial of an antidepressant.

INVESTIGATIONS

Since dementia is a clinical syndrome and not a disease, full investigation is required for each patient. Much information is obtained from a careful history of the patient and from partner or family members. An assessment of the pattern of the cognitive impairment, both by bedside testing and more detailed assessment of neuropsychological function, will provide the likely diagnosis in the majority of cases. Neuroimaging or brain scan, of which magnetic resonance imaging (MRI) is the most useful, will exclude many of the secondary causes of dementia such as tumors and strokes. A variety of blood tests and occasionally an electroencephalogram (EEG) will complete the investigation. Some patients will require more intensive investigation such as examination of the cerebrospinal fluid.

The majority of patients will have an underlying degenerative disease, whether it is Alzheimer's disease, frontotemporal dementia, or dementia with Lewy bodies. As such, many of the investigations are essentially normal, but this can be difficult for the patient and family to understand. Normal means that many other abnormalities have been excluded. Neither brain scan nor the other investigations can provide a definitive diagnosis of the underlying degenerative disease. This can only be established with certainty by examination of brain tissue. However, with careful clinical assessment, supplemented by investigations, a diagnosis can be made with approximately 80 percent accuracy. The 20 percent of uncertainty tends to be in identifying other degenerative diseases rather than missing a major reversible cause. Increasingly, MRI scans can demonstrate tissue loss, which is common among degenerative diseases, and in a characteristic distribution, as in FTD.

Finally, it is important to remember that our classification of diseases is there to help manage patients. We classify patients and their problems either at the level of the clinical presentations (memory impairment or dementia); damage to an organ (frontotemporal lobar degeneration or strokes); or at a molecular level, in terms of specific DNA mutations in familial disease or particular abnormal proteins that are deposited.

Which classification we choose to use when we determine that changes in cognition are abnormal is determined by what is helpful to us as clinicians and patients to manage these distressing problems.

Table I. Frontotemporal Dementia and Alzheimer's Disease: Similarities and Differences		
Features	Frontotemporal Dementia	Alzheimer's Disease
Age at which disease generally occurs	• common between 40 and 70 years	• Common in the eldery
Brain areas affected	• frontal and temporal lobes	• starts in the medial temporal area, usually in the hippocampus • spreads to other areas of the brain
Pathologic features	• loss of nerve cells • no amyloid plaques • tau protein tangles seen in certain FTDs, but different from AD tangles	• loss of nerve cells • amyloid plaques • tau tangles
Clinical features	• varying personality and behavior changes, from apathy to hyperactivity • loss of empathy toward others; lack of proper social conduct • memory is preserved early on • language difficulty • compulsive eating and oral fixations • repetitive actions	• begins with memory loss • loss of ability to learn new information • inability to orient oneself to time and place • later, personality and behavior problems develop • possible hallucinations and delusions in later stages

CHAPTER 2

What Is Frontotemporal Dementia?
A Clinical Perspective

MURRAY GROSSMAN

INTRODUCTION

FTD is a progressive neurodegenerative condition that typically begins in the fifth or sixth decade of life, although cases have been reported with an onset as young as twenty-one years of age and as old as eigty-five years of age. FTD differs from AD in that the frequency of AD, but not FTD, increases with age. There are many other features that distinguish between FTD and AD as well, and these will be noted below when the clinical features of FTD are described. There do not appear to be any geographic or sociodemographic risk factors associated with FTD. There is no evidence that head trauma or consumption of a particular food is a risk factor for the development of FTD. There have been no epidemiologic studies that are community-based to establish the frequency of this condition in the population, although we know that FTD is relatively uncommon in comparison to AD and Parkinson's disease. However, estimates suggest that between 2 and 13 percent of autopsy series of demented patients in large hospitals have FTD or a related disorder. In large clinics, the estimated frequency of FTD ranges from 5 to 20 percent. Perhaps the most common etiology of FTD is Dementia Lacking Distinctive Histopathology. Other conditions causing FTD include Pick's disease, corticobasal degeneration, frontotemporal dementia with Parkinsonism associated with a defect on chromo-

41

some 17 (FTDP-17), very unusual presentations of Alzheimer's disease, FTD-associated motor neuron disease, and a large number of very unusual and rare diseases.

This chapter focuses on the clinical features of FTD. The first discussion will be the major clinical presentations, including changes in cognition, language, and affect. Some of the neurological changes associated with FTD also will be described. Following a description of these initial clinical presentations, the natural history, prognosis, and diagnosis of this condition will be addressed.

CLINICAL PRESENTATION

The Syndromic Approach to Frontotemporal Dementia

FTD typically presents with one of two clinical syndromes, although there are some less common presentations that will be mentioned below as well. Two clinical presentations are particularly common. These include: progressive aphasia, and a disorder of social comportment and behavior. Less commonly documented are presentations involving a motor-speech disorder known as dysarthria, an isolated dysexecutive syndrome involving poor planning and organization, and a disorder of visual-perceptual-spatial functioning.

Progressive Aphasia

Aphasia is a central disorder of speech and language—there is no deafness, blindness, or muteness due to motor weakness—that can affect oral and written comprehension and production. Components of language can be impaired in isolation or in combination with other language processes, depending on the portion of the brain that is compromised in FTD. One form of aphasia is Progressive Fluent Aphasia. This is also known as Semantic Dementia. The dominant clinical feature of this presentation is difficulty in the comprehension of single words and the use of single words to name objects. These patients will have difficulty recognizing even highly frequent single words and will express confusion when they are heard. The difficulty with single-word comprehension may begin with isolated vocabulary terms, but will gradually involve larger portions of the vocabulary over time. A (lost) word will not be able to be described by semantic dementia patients except in the most vague manner. Difficulty with single-word comprehension and retrieval will be evident in both oral communication and writing. For other terms where there is an isolated anomia or naming difficulty, patients will attempt to describe the intended target in a circumlocutory manner by talking around the target word. Difficulty with reading may be most pronounced for sight vocabulary terms that cannot be sounded out, such as "who" or "choir." Similarly, patients may have more difficulty spelling sight vocabulary terms orally and in writing compared to words that obey letter-sound correspondence rules. Speech remains relatively fluent in these patients, sentence production is grammatically well formed, and comprehension of grammar appears to be preserved.

Another form of language difficulty commonly seen in FTD is Progressive Nonfluent Aphasia (PNFA). In this form of progressive aphasia, comprehension and expression of single words is relatively preserved, although these patients do have some naming difficulty. Instead, the major problem is concerned with speech fluency. This depends on the patient's access to grammatical forms such as the small grammatical words that allow us to construct a sentence. Without these grammatical components, speech is disjointed and effortful. Oral and written utterances consist largely of slowly produced content words. Comprehension is similarly affected. Progressive nonfluent aphasics thus have difficulty determining who did what to whom in a sentence.

A less common form of progressive aphasia affects predominantly the motor speech apparatus and causes a progressive form of dysarthria (poorly articulated speech). Sometimes this is called speech apraxia. In patients with progressive dysarthria, comprehension is preserved and expression is grammatical. However, speech is garbled. There is no evidence for primary motor weakness of the face muscles or tongue, but the coordinated functioning of the orofacial motor apparatus appears to be impaired. There is no difficulty with reading or writing in this condition, although oral reading can sound the same as spontaneous speech. Unusual cases of isolated reading difficulty (progressive alexia) and writing difficulty (progressive agraphia) have been reported, but these are extremely rare.

Disorders of Affect and Social Comportment

Another major clinical presentation of FTD involves a disorder of mood, affect, and social comportment. These patients are noteworthy for inappropriate social conduct that seems insensitive to the norms governing social interactions and personal behavior in society. Initially, these patients appear to make some odd or inappropriate statements or voice unusual opinions. Over a short period of time, however, it becomes clear that this approach to social interactions is not restricted to a single event but reflects a broad sense of inappropriateness. These patients lack empathy for difficulties that others may be encountering. This lack of empathy is not restricted to strangers but also involves spouses and other family members with whom there is great familiarity and intimacy. Comments emerge that are disinhibited and may be blurted out without any sensitivity or consideration of context. There is a loss of social graces and a frank rudeness that may be quite out of line with the patient's premorbid personality. There appears to be little insight into the intentions of others, and the patients may appear to be entirely self-centered.

This stark change in personality can have consequences in other domains. Patients can appear to be hypersexual. This can manifest itself as promiscuous sexual encounters with strangers or inappropriate and unsatisfied sexual demands of spouses. Subtler manifestations of hypersexual behavior may include a fetish associated with a movie star, a focus on sexual jokes, and inappropriate sexual comments that seem disinhibited and out of context.

Another form of disinhibited behavior can involve an inappropriate attraction to small shiny objects or fire. At times this can be manifested as shoplifting or pocketing attractive artifacts from friends' houses.

Inappropriate rage responses also can be seen in these patients. This involves sudden, unexpected outbursts of angry behavior that rarely can become violent. The provocation can be minimal or even imagined in nature. Regardless of the perceived slight, these patients can produce a verbal tirade that sometimes can be difficult to quell. The patients do not appear to understand the reason for physical restraint.

Hyperoral behavior can be quite common in these patients. This can range from the disinhibited consumption of large volumes of food to oral exploration of inedible objects. Obsessive changes in dietary preferences can emerge and the diet may become restricted to highly idiosyncratic choices of substances. These changes in oral behavior can be accompanied by radical changes in weight.

There can be important changes in motivation. Patients may appear to be profoundly apathetic. They have difficulty initiating the simplest behaviors spontaneously. Even significant prompting by a loved one for participation in a previously enjoyed hobby or avocation can yield no response. Patients may be content to literally do nothing all day. This disorder of motivation and apathy can affect all realms of human behavior, resulting in an akinetic state or mutism. Incontinence may emerge early in this context because of limited motivation to use the bathroom.

Dysexecutive Syndrome

A form of cognitive difficulty overlapping with progressive aphasia and social disorder is a limitation in executive functioning. Executive resources include selective attention and control over inhibition, task switching, and planning and organizing. Difficulties with control over attention and inhibition can emerge as perseveration or repeatedly performing the same activities. This can also be manifested as echolalia or mindlessly repeating a phrase that has just been uttered. Echopraxia, or mindlessly repeating a gesture, also can be seen. Patients are distracted quite easily and can have difficulty refocusing their attention. Patients also can become environmentally dependent or perceptually bound. This involves thoughtlessly incorporating objects in the environment into ongoing activities.

Task switching involves the ability to alternate between ongoing cognitive or physical activities in a flexible and organized manner. This can limit productive behavior since performance is restricted to the execution of simple tasks. Each new event or thought has to be initiated anew, and patients consequently can appear to be quite sluggish and slow in their performance of activities, including familiar activities of daily living. Considerable guidance is needed, even for overlearned activities such as bathing.

Working memory involves the ability to manipulate a relatively small amount of information held in short-term memory over a brief period of time. Working memory is involved in a large number of ongoing cognitive activities such as the comprehension of a conversation or a movie. Limitations in working memory can result in the appearance of disjointedness in the course of a conversation, and poor working memory can result in reduced enjoyment of previously appreciated activities such as watching TV or reading a book.

Activities in our complex society often require planning and organizing. This may be the heart of the concept of executive resources, and includes activities such as performing two tasks at once. In this context, patients can execute complex activities when guided by others or constrained by the environment. When performing activities spontaneously and without constraint, however, the patients can appear remarkably impaired. This can result in the phenomenon of a patient being quite incapacitated in the performance of activities in the world, without evidence for difficulties during a highly constrained medical or psychiatric examination.

Unusual Clinical Manifestations of FTD

A handful of unusual presentations of FTD have come to medical attention and have been associated with FTD as a result of autopsy confirmation of the diagnosis. Some patients can present predominantly with visual-spatial-perceptual impairments. A handful of patients have been described with a form of visual agnosia or difficulty comprehending seen objects. Patients may be able to identify individual attributes of a visual array such as the color or the size of an object. However, they cannot assemble this fragmented information into a coherent whole. Organizational difficulties may be limited to the visual domain. A small number of patients have been described with limb apraxia or difficulty executing learned motor skills. Oftentimes these are involved in the inappropriate use of implements. A tool may be held in the wrong way or may be used at the wrong angle. Under rare circumstances, gestures may not be understood.

Corticobasal degeneration (CBD) is another rare condition allied to FTD. Early descriptions of CBD often emphasized the movement disorders associated with the condition, such as gait instability, body stiffness, brief and lightning-like movements known as myoclonus, and an impairment using limbs in a meaningful manner (so-called

Alien Hand syndrome). More recently, it has become clear that CBD patients often have predominantly cognitive difficulties. These include problems with naming, visual-perceptual-spatial functioning, apraxia, calculation difficulty, and an impairment interpreting the meaning of objects that are palpated (so-called cortical sensory loss).

Natural History

FTD is a progressive neurodegenerative condition, and patients will worsen over time in the cognitive domains where they have difficulty. The trajectory of decline over time, however, is not linear. Instead, there appears to be a biphasic change over time. Specifically, during the initial or mild stage of FTD, there can be a relatively prolonged period of subtle but insidious change that involves few fundamental differences. The subtle changes that do emerge over time are typically restricted to the domain of difficulty that brought the patient to medical attention in the first place. For example, there may be subtle and progressive decline in single-word comprehension and vocabulary in patients with semantic dementia. Patients with progressive nonfluent aphasia can have increasing difficulty with grammatical comprehension and expression. Patients with a disorder of personality and social comportment can have gradually worsening behavior. It is only under very unusual circumstances that progressive change evolves rapidly during the early course of FTD, and a rapid change should call to question the diagnosis. Similarly, the absence of change over a prolonged period of time should also raise questions about the underlying diagnosis.

The second or moderate stage of FTD involves a more rapidly emerging series of changes over a briefer time course. During this phase of the condition, qualitatively different kinds of language, cognitive, and behavioral changes can emerge. For example, a patient presenting with semantic dementia can begin having difficulty with grammatical aspects of language. A progressive nonfluent aphasic can begin to demonstrate personality and social changes. A patient with a disorder of social comportment can begin to demonstrate executive limitations.

At a functional level, patients in the moderate stage of FTD become increasingly dependent on others for instrumental activities of daily living. This can involve increasing dependence on others for day-to-day care activities, such as grooming and dressing, that previously may have been performed independently. Patients may require verbal guidance and prompting to perform activities such as bathing.

The severe stage of FTD is characterized functionally by dependence on others for virtually all activities of daily living. This can include toileting, feeding, and basic mobility. Language, cognitive, and personality disorders can be quite broad based.

In the severe stage of disease, because patients are quite dependent on others for daily needs, there is increased risk of morbidity and mortality associated with meeting these needs. One example is that difficulty with independent feeding can result in aspiration of food into the lungs. This can cause chemical pneumonia, a frequent cause of death among FTD patients. The issues leading to aspiration are multifactorial. There can be difficulty coordinating the orofacial musculature. Patients can also be easily distracted from concentrating on a fundamental activity that previously had been automatic. For example, attention is needed to swallow food in a safe manner. Patients also may not appreciate the need to swallow, and instead can continue to place food in the mouth in an unregulated manner.

Another example of morbidity in the severe stage of FTD is concerned with the role of mobility and frequent postural adjustments to avoid decubitus ulcers or skin breakdown in the form of bedsores. As part of normal mobility, we frequently adjust our posture so that our body's weight does not rest for long periods of time on the same portions of our skin. In apathetic patients with reduced motivation and limited planning, there may be long periods of time where they do not adjust posture and remain dependent on the same portions of skin. This limits blood circulation to the area and causes death to skin tissue. Skin breakdown results in infection that can spread to the bloodstream.

Patients with FTD can become incontinent quite early in the course of their condition because of apathy and poor motivation associated with poor social insight. Incontinence can be associated with infection. Urinary tract infections can develop, particularly in women, that can spread to the kidneys and bloodstream if not treated appropriately.

Prognosis

The time course over which these changes evolve can be quite variable and is difficult to predict. Under rare circumstances, there can be relatively rapid decline over the course of eighteen to twenty-four months. This form of FTD is often associated with motor neuron disease. Even under more common circumstances, the natural history of FTD can be quite varied. Some clinical impressions are that younger patients tend to progress more rapidly, although there are no data to support this observation. In this younger cohort of FTD patients, the prognosis can evolve over four or five years. On the other hand, the natural history can be quite prolonged in some individuals, particularly where there are no other health related co-morbidities.

There are additional neurological changes that can have a negative impact on prognosis. One relatively common change is concerned with gait. Changes in balance and gait stability can result in frequent falls. This may be due in part to poor postural adjustment associated with axial rigidity. Frequent falls increase the risk for fractures of the hip, vertebrae, or skull that can have profound and wide ranging consequences. In addition, patients can develop a subdural hematoma, a collection of blood between the brain and the skull that can result from closed head injury.

Other neurological changes that can contribute to a poor prognosis include lateralized weakness of the face or a limb. Although rare, features of Parkinsonism, such as tremor, can emerge. Disorders of visual acuity are not known to be associated with FTD, and disorders of eye movements are oftentimes associated with specific neurodegenerative diseases that are not FTD. Despite common language difficulty, deficits in auditory acuity are not known to occur in FTD. Weakness of the neck and tongue muscles can be seen in motor neuron disease associated with FTD, but this is a relatively uncommon syndrome. Clumsiness—inaccurately reaching for an object or walking with a wide-based gait—is not associated with FTD. A disorder of sensation, such as reduced sensitivity to touch or temperature, should raise concern about another disorder.

MEDICAL INVESTIGATIONS

A variety of disorders can mimic FTD. It is important to detect these because some are treatable. Serum studies looking for B_{12} deficiency, reduced thyroid functioning, and other age-related disorders of metabolism should be performed. Under unusual circumstances, inflammation of the small arteries bringing blood to the brain can result in microscopically sized areas of ischemia or stroke. These can interfere with brain functioning, despite the absence of gross neurologic changes associated with larger strokes.

There also are a variety of infections producing cognitive changes that can emerge over a more prolonged period of time than is typically associated with meningoencephalitis. The detection of some kinds of infection can be made reliably only with a lumbar puncture, required for examination of the cerebrospinal fluid bathing the brain and spinal cord.

Unusual forms of partial-complex seizure activity can mimic FTD in some circumstances. This may be detected only with a careful history and an EEG.

A structural image of the brain is necessary to rule out several conditions that can mimic FTD. For example, the accumulation of small strokes oftentimes can be detected only by MRI. Similarly, subtle forms of hydrocephalus require exclusion by MRI and possibly lumbar puncture. Other conditions that can potentially mimic FTD also can be excluded by MRI, including closed head injury, subdural hematoma, and a brain tumor or other forms of cancer. FTD itself is associated at times with focal atrophy or shrinkage of brain regions such as the frontal and temporal lobes of the brain.

Oftentimes the panel of medical investigations is within normal limits and atrophy on MRI is too subtle to provide reliable confirmation of a diagnosis of FTD. Under these circumstances, a functional neuroimaging study such as a Positron Emission Tomography (PET) scan or a Single Proton Emission Computed Tomography (SPECT) scan can be quite useful. New forms of functional MRI are being developed that are very sensitive to deficits in brain activity. These investigations can demonstrate focal reductions in gray matter functioning in an anatomic distribution of the brain that corresponds to the patient's clinical difficulties. While several experimental procedures for diagnosing FTD are currently under development, there is no known definitive diagnostic test for FTD short of the direct examination of the brain with a biopsy or at autopsy. In chapter 8 the diagnostic criteria for FTD based on neuropathology findings are presented.

Based on clinical presentations discussed earlier in this chapter, exclusion of other disorders that can mimic FTD, and use of neuroimaging studies, a clinician can recognize and diagnosis FTD. Since there is no definitive test that is easily obtainable in a living patient, clinical criteria for FTD have been established to help guide physicians. (See table 1.)

TREATMENT AND MANAGEMENT

Treatment and management of FTD is in its infancy. There have been few systematic clinical trials of medications or observations of behavioral interventions that have been well studied. In this context, management and treatment often is based on rational approaches derived from the principles of medical therapeutics. These issues are addressed in detail elsewhere in this book. Common sense safety precautions for the patient and the family should be implemented, and these are described in part 2 of this book.

Symptomatic treatment can take the form of neurotransmitter supplementation. Medications borrowed from other conditions— such as Alzheimer's disease, Parkinson's disease, and depression— can contribute to clinical slowing of progression. Other symptomatic treatments are directed at specific complaints, such as the treatment of hallucinations, depression, fatigue, anxiety, and hypersexual behavior. Other substances that may alter the natural history of FTD include antioxidants such as vitamin E, and nonsteroidal anti-inflammatory agents. It is important to discuss medications with a physician before initiating a treatment trial.

There are also behavioral interventions that may be beneficial. There is very reasonable evidence supporting the claim that physical activity and mental activity are quite beneficial. Indeed, some evidence suggests a synergistic relationship between physical and mental activity that, when performed daily, is more beneficial than the sum of each.

SUMMARY

The care of patients with frontotemporal dementia is demanding on families and friends. Some of this burden can be eased with better understanding of the condition. The goal of this chapter was to characterize FTD in a manner that will familiarize families and friends with some of the clinical features of this condition. This should help explain previous experiences that may have been misinterpreted, such as understanding that unusual behavior is not willful but is a component of the disease process. Moreover, it is important to be able to understand what the future may hold. Also, this chapter helps one appreciate the complexity of diagnosis for this group of conditions through an understanding of the various clinical presentations and lack of a specific diagnostic test. As this group of conditions has only recently been defined there is more research needed to determine the underlying cause or biology along with treatment and management.

Table I. Clinical Criteria for FTD[1]

The following criteria were established at an international conference in July 2000, which brought together clinicians and basic scientists with expertise in frontotemporal dementia. The purpose of these criteria is to aid neurologists, psychiatrists, and other healthcare providers in recognizing FTD. At this same meeting diagnostic criteria for FTD based on neuropathology studies also were established. (See chapter 8.)

1. The development of behavioral or cognitive deficits is demonstrated by

    - early onset and progressive change in personality, characterized by difficulty in controlling or changing behavior, often resulting in inappropriate responses or activities (disorders of affect and social comportment), or
    - early onset and progressive change in language, characterized by problems with expression of language or severe naming difficulty and problems with word meaning (progressive aphasia).

2. The deficits outlined above cause significant impairment in social or occupational functioning and represent a significant decline from a previous level of functioning.

3. The course is characterized by a gradual onset and continuing decline in function.

4. The deficits outlined above are not due to other nervous system conditions (e.g., stroke), systemic conditions (e.g., thyroid disease), or substance-induced conditions.

5. The deficits do not occur exclusively during a delirium.

6. The disturbance is not better accounted for by a psychiatric diagnosis (e.g., depression).

NOTES

This work was supported in part by grants from the United States Public Health Service (AG 17586, AG 15116, and NS 35867). This work would not have been possible without the support of the patients and the families for whom I care. Their strength and insight continually overwhelm me.
    1. G. M. McKhann et al., "Clinical and pathological diagnosis of frontotemporal dementias: Report of the work group on frontotemporal dementia and Pick's disease," *Archives of Neurology* 58 (June 2001): 1803–1806.

CHAPTER 3

The Role of Genetics:

A Piece in the FTD Puzzle

JENNIFER M. FARMER

I t was once thought that genetics pertained only to very rare diseases, often affecting children. Now we are constantly reminded that genetics has a much more prominent and complex role in common conditions such as cancer, diabetes, and Alzheimer's disease. The media routinely provides the public with information about the identification of genes linked to diseases and encourages individuals to pay attention to their family medical history. Also, as researchers struggle to learn about the underlying causes of specific conditions, they are looking more and more to genetics. This is true for frontotemporal dementia. As researchers try to determine what causes FTD, some are actively engaged in attempts to identify specific genes that are linked to it. By understanding genetics, one can learn more about the biological basis of the condition, and this knowledge can be used to investigate novel treatments.

The goals of this chapter include:

- explaining the importance of obtaining family history information
- providing a brief introduction to genetics and patterns of inheritance
- discussing the genetics of FTD
- reviewing the utility and goals of genetic testing and genetic counseling

OBTAINING A FAMILY MEDICAL HISTORY

When a physician or healthcare provider is evaluating a patient for a diagnosis of FTD or similar neurodegenerative condition, information regarding the family history can help determine a diagnosis. Thus, a detailed family history is a valuable diagnostic tool. It is worth the time and effort to contact relatives and obtain the most accurate details of family structure and medical information. A complete family history that describes structure and health history contains a lot of information. It is important to document the information in a meaningful way that is accessible and easy to read. Geneticists and genetic counselors create a pedigree, which is a graphic description of family structure and health history, to record information collected from patients and families. Determining the quantity and quality of information to collect can be difficult. It is generally recommended to research at least three generations of relatives, which includes:

- first-degree relatives
  —children, siblings, and parents
- second-degree relatives
  —half-siblings, aunts, uncles, nieces, nephews, grandparents, grandchildren
- third-degree relatives
  —cousins

The type of medical information to obtain on relatives can include:

- vital status (living or deceased)
  —age (date of birth)
  —age of death
  —cause of death
  —autopsy
- pregnancy, miscarriages, and stillborns
- infertility
- individuals with previous genetics evaluation
- environmental exposures
  —radiation, alcohol or drug abuse, tobacco
- health history
  —birth defects
  —mental retardation
  —deafness, blindness
  —chronic childhood illness
  —cancer
  —neurological conditions (e.g., epilepsy, migraines, strokes, multiple sclerosis, Parkinson's disease)
  —mental illness (e.g., bipolar disorder, schizophrenia, OCD)
  —dementia (Alzheimer's disease, senility)
- ages of diagnoses

When going back and obtaining medical information from previous generations, keep in mind that many of the medical terms we use today, such as FTD and corticalbasal degeneration, were previously not used. Therefore, many individuals with neurodegenerative conditions would have been told that they had dementia or senility. In such cases, it can be useful to try to gather more descriptive information. For example, it is useful to ask if the individual had problems speaking as a first symptom, or if he had a personality or behavior change. It is also important to try to determine an estimate for the age of onset. Another way to determine diagnosis in deceased relatives is to inquire about autopsy. If an individual had an autopsy, oftentimes the autopsy records (as well as other records, MRI reports, and brain biopsies) can be requested. These records can be most informative. Confirmation of diagnoses with medical records from previous evaluations and laboratory studies is also crucial.

The family medical history or pedigree can be a powerful diagnostic tool to a clinician evaluating a patient. The pedigree can be utilized as a diagnostic tool in the following ways:

- establish pattern of inheritance
- identify individuals in the family who are at risk for the condition
- determine strategies for genetic testing
- help screen for medical risks (such as cancer and heart disease)

Family history information needs to be respected and treated appropriately by healthcare providers and individual family members. Contacting relatives and asking about personal information is not an easy task. Navigating through the complex interpersonal relationships and personalities in a family can be emotionally difficult and stressful. This is a give-and-take process; it is important to state your intentions or reasons for collecting the information. Offer to re-contact family members with information that you learn about your loved one's diagnosis and how it may affect them. Respect an individual's right to privacy. If you go through the effort of obtaining a family history, be sure to document the information clearly and secure it in a location that is accessible to other family members and future generations.

INTRODUCTION TO GENETICS AND INHERITANCE

Deoxyribonucleic acid (DNA) is a chemical that is the most basic unit of genetic information. Chromosomes are highly organized structures containing DNA in long strands. (See figure 1.) Most cells in our body contain a complete set of forty-six chromosomes, or twenty-three pairs. The chromosomes are numbered 1 to 22 (largest to smallest) and the twenty-third pair are the sex chromosomes, which determine gender (two X chromosomes = female or one X and one Y chromosome = male). We inherit our chromosomes at the time of conception: one set of twenty-three from our mother and one set of twenty-three from our father. As we grow from a single cell into a complex human being, our chromosomes are copied into each new cell. Genes are specific subunits or groups of DNA along the chromosomes. Just as our chromosomes come in pairs, so do our genes. Each gene codes for a protein (or chemical) that has a specific function in the body.

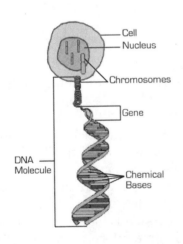

Figure 1: This is an illustration of DNA, chromosomes, and genes, which are discussed in the text. (From National Cancer Institute, Understanding Gene Testing, http://newscenter. cancer.gov/sciencebehind/genetesting/genetesting/00.htm)

The following analogy can be illustrative. One can think of a gene as a long word. Every letter in the word is a piece of DNA. Just like words, genes must be "spelled" or have the correct DNA code to function properly. There are two types of misspellings that can occur in our DNA. One type includes words with multiple spellings but with the same meaning or a misspelling that is silent and allows the word to still be read correctly. For example, the word "theater" is sometimes spelled as "theatre." Despite this alteration, you still understand the word and its meaning. This type of alteration in the DNA code is called a polymorphism. The second type of misspelling involves changes to the word that alter the meaning or make the word unreadable. For example, if the word "good" were changed to "gxod," one would not be able to make sense out of "gxod." This type of misspelling or change in the DNA code is called a mutation. Mutations alter the function of the gene and are often associated with disease.

Inherited conditions can be passed on in families in different ways. Autosomal dominant conditions affect males and females equally and only one gene of the pair needs to be abnormal for the individual to have the condition. Autosomal dominant conditions are passed from an affected individual to offspring with a 50 percent chance. (See figure 2.) The word "autosomal" means the gene that causes the condition is on a numbered chromosome (1 to 22), not one of the sex chromosomes (X or Y). When examining a family history for an autosomal dominant condition, oftentimes one will identify multiple individuals in each generation with the condition. If an individual did not inherit the abnormal gene, then she cannot pass it on.

Autosomal recessive conditions affect males and females equally, but both copies of the disease gene need to be abnormal for the individual to have the condition. Autosomal recessive conditions can be passed on when each parent is a carrier for the condition, and their offspring have a 25 percent risk of inheriting the condition. (See figure 3.) Carriers have one abnormal copy of the gene but do not have clinical symptoms and are not at increased risk to develop the

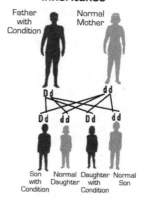

Autosomal Dominant Inheritance

Figure 2: Features of autosomal dominant inheritance. The condition appears in multiple individuals, in successive generations, and each affected individual has an affected parent. Any offspring of an affected parent has a 50 percent risk of inheriting the condition. Nonaffected individuals do not transmit the condition to offspring. Males and females are equally likely to have the condition.

Autosomal Recessive Inheritance

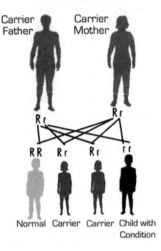

Figure 3: Features of autosomal recessive inheritance. The condition appears in multiple members of sibship, not in the parents or offspring. If the family is small there may only be one affected individual. The recurrence risk for each sibling is 25 percent. Males and females are equally likely to have the condition. Parents may be consanguineous (related).

condition. A family history of a recessive condition can reveal multiple individuals in a single generation (brothers and sisters) with the condition or, in the case of small families, there may be no other affected individuals. Autosomal recessive conditions also appear more frequently among individuals with the same ethnic background or among individuals who marry within the same family. Other types of inheritance include conditions that are linked to the sex chromosomes (X-linked) or those that are only passed on through maternal transmission.

Based on genetic research, we now appreciate that not all genetic conditions are caused by a single gene and show a clear pattern of inheritance when one examines the family tree. Rather, many conditions, especially neurodegenerative conditions, are caused by changes in multiple genes that create a susceptibility or increased risk for the condition, combined with environmental influences (e.g., head trauma, infection). Conditions that are caused by both genetic and environmental influences are called multifactorial. Often, multifactorial conditions are seen in multiple family members but without a specific pattern to the inheritance. However, these conditions can also appear in one individual. Understanding the genetic contributions to multifactorial conditions can be useful to researchers in trying to identify treatments. Also, knowledge of the genetics can help individuals learn more about their risk for developing a condition.

GENETICS OF FTD

About 30 percent of individuals with FTD do have other family members with a neurodegenerative condition or dementia. However, fewer (approximately 10 percent) families with a strong history of an FTD-like condition pass on the disorder in an autosomal dominant fashion. FTD, Pick's disease, Alzheimer's disease, or dementia are described among first-degree relatives in multiple generations. Individuals diagnosed with FTD who do not have a family history of the disorder or other neurodegenerative conditions are referred to as sporadic, which is used to describe the lack of an inherited influence. In cases of familial or inherited FTD, the age of onset is often younger than those with sporadic presentations (twenties, thirties, and forties for familial FTD), and it is not uncommon for the condition to progress more rapidly.

Researchers have been collecting blood and tissue samples from individuals with suggestive familial FTD and related conditions to try to determine the specific genetic cause for this group of diseases. This has lead to the identification of the *MAPT* gene on chromosome 17, which codes for the protein called tau. Abnormal amounts of tau have been described in neuropathology (brain tissue) and cerebrospinal fluid (fluid that surrounds the brain) investigations among individuals with FTD, Alzheimer's disease, and other neurodegenerative conditions. For more detailed information about the role of tau in pathology and brain cells, refer to chapter 8.

The families that were originally linked to the *MAPT* gene (commonly referred to as tau) were given a more specific diagnosis called frontotemporal dementia with Parkinsonism (FTPD-17). This condition was clinically described by the presence of dementia and/or Parkinsonism, frontal and/or temporal atrophy of the brain, as well as two or more similarly affected family members consistent with an autosomal dominant pattern of inheritance. About 25 to 40 percent of families with autosomal dominant inheritance of FTD (or similar condition) have mutations in the *MAPT* gene. This means that other genes are likely to be identified and implicated in causing FTD. There have been reports of possible familial FTD linkage to a region on chromosome 3, but no disease-associated gene has been identified.

More than fifty families have been found to have mutations in the *MAPT* gene. Many of these families have unique mutations that have only been described once. However, there are a few mutations that have been seen in multiple families around the world. In such cases, where the same mutation is seen in different families, specific phenotypic (clinical) features have been compared. These types of studies are called genotype/phenotype correlations. Such information can be useful for counseling families about the associated clinical findings and prognosis when a known mutation is identified. For example, some mutations are associated with a more rapid progression of the condition. There has also been a mutation identified in a family with a form of FTD that includes motor neuron disease or ALS (Lou Gehrig's disease).

Many polymorphisms have been described in the *MAPT* gene that are not directly linked to disease, although there are some specific patterns of polymorphisms, called "haplotypes," that have been implicated by association with FTD. Researchers are trying to determine how specific haplotypes may modify risk for FTD. Studies of individuals with sporadic FTD have not yielded mutations in the *MAPT* gene.

In the future, genetic research will:

- discover more mutations in the *MAPT* gene and therefore the clinical features associated with FTDP-17 will expand
- identify genotype/phenotype correlations that will be useful in providing genetic counseling to families
- find novel FTD-associated genes that will help researchers understand the cause and biology of the FTDs

GENETIC COUNSELING AND GENETIC TESTING

Genetic counseling is a communication process between an individual (or the family) and a healthcare provider with special training in genetics. Some of the activities in a typical genetic counseling session are:

- construction of a pedigree and analysis for patterns of inheritance and genetic risk

- education about natural history, genetics, and inheritance of condition
- discussion of recurrence risk for inherited and multifactorial conditions
- discussion of benefits and limitations of genetic testing
- psychosocial support for individuals and families coping with a diagnosis

A genetic counselor can also be an important ally in advocating healthcare needs for patients and families.

Genetic testing can be extremely complex. Not all tests are 100 percent diagnostic, and often there are ethical and social concerns that influence one's decision to have or not to have genetic testing. Genetic testing for FTD has been offered on a research basis mostly to individuals with a suspected familial FTD. There is an important distinction between research-based genetic testing and clinical or commercial genetic testing. Research testing is not a diagnostic test. There is no guarantee of a result that will be of benefit to the patient. Usually the goal of research testing is to advance scientific knowledge about the condition. This research is usually conducted in academic laboratories. A study coordinator or physician should review the details of the study and obtain informed consent from the patient and/or family members for participation. You should be provided with an informed consent form that has been approved by an Institutional Review Board (IRB) at the university or hospital where the research is being performed. Clinical or commercial genetic testing is a diagnostic test. The patient receives an official result from the test. The testing is performed in a laboratory that has been approved for this type of diagnostic testing to insure the integrity of the results. Such laboratories are located in hospitals, universities, biotechnology companies, and commercial laboratories. Often, clinical genetic testing is offered only after the patient and family have received genetic counseling to explore the benefits and limitations of testing.

In the near future clinical genetic testing will be available for diagnosis of individuals with or at risk for FTD. However, this test will not be useful to all individuals. For example, genetic testing to identify disease-associated mutations in the *MAPT* gene will only be recommended to individuals with a dominant family history of

FTD, and this testing will most likely identify mutations in about 25 to 40 percent of individuals. As more causative genes for FTD are identified, research testing will move to the clinical arena, further expanding the role of genetic testing for diagnosis of FTD.

Many individuals who are presently asymptomatic, but believe that they are at increased risk for FTD based on family history, have expressed an interest in genetic testing so that they can learn if they inherited the gene. Presymptomatic or predisposition genetic testing is not a new concept in coping with neurodegenerative conditions. Such testing has been offered to individuals at risk for Huntington's disease, familial Alzheimer's disease, and other genetic conditions. For the vast majority of these conditions, FTD included, there is no treatment. Therefore an individual who has the presymptomatic genetic testing may learn that he is destined to have a progressive, debilitating disease. Genetic counseling for the at-risk individual is paramount. Many clinical centers and laboratories require that the individual go through a formal protocol of pre- and post-test genetic counseling along with psychiatric evaluation. This offers the individual an opportunity to discuss his motives for testing; explore the possible result outcomes, anticipated reaction, and coping strategies; develop a support system; and discuss the risks associated with receiving a diagnosis (such as adverse psychological outcome and insurance or employment discrimination). Also, it is important to have the specific genetic abnormality or mutation in an affected family member documented to confirm the diagnosis before testing at-risk individuals. If a genetic mutation is not known in the affected family member, testing in other relatives has a great risk of being uninformative. Genetic testing for untreatable conditions is not recommended for at-risk children because they are not able to provide informed consent, and giving a child a label may do great harm.

Genetic counselors have master's level training in human or medical genetics or genetic counseling and are certified by the American Board of Genetic Counseling. To locate a genetic counselor, inquire at your local medical center or contact the National Society of Genetic Counselors via the internet at www.nsgc.org and go to the Resource link to identify someone near you.

CONCLUSION

Genetics is a crucial piece of the FTD puzzle. There are more FTD-associated genes to be revealed and applied to the pathophysiology. To determine the cause of sporadic FTD, there is a great challenge to understand the complex interactions of genetic, environmental, and pathological factors. Genetic testing continues to improve and will prove to be a valuable diagnostic tool for more families and individuals with FTD. Genetic counseling is essential to help identify and accurately interpret risk, provide education, and explore the benefits and limitations of genetic testing.

RESOURCES

Genetic Alliance, Inc.—www.geneticalliance.org
    The alliance supports individuals with genetic conditions and their families, educates the public, and advocates for consumer-informed public policies.

National Human Genome Research Institute—www.genome.gov
    The National Human Genome Research Institute leads the Human Genome Project for the National Institutes of Health, conducts cutting-edge research in its laboratories, and supports genomic science worldwide. This Web site contains a lot of useful information for the layperson about the human genome project, genetic research, and genetic conditions and testing.

National Society of Genetic Counselors, Inc.—www.nsgc.org
    Go to the Resource link to find a genetic counselor.

CHAPTER 4

Finding the "A" Team:

Creating a Collaboration of Health Professionals

CAROL F. LIPPA

Identifying the right physician or healthcare team can be a challenging experience regardless of the underlying medical condition. The situation is even more complicated when there are specialized needs because an individual has a cognitive or behavioral disorder. FTD patients seldom have the insight to seek medical help on their own. Many would deny a problem even if their physician brought up the issue. For this reason, they are usually brought to medical attention by a caregiver. The caregiver needs to find the right physician and then persuade the often unwilling individual to be assessed by the healthcare team. This can be one of the hardest things a caregiver has to do. Due to the reluctance of many FTD patients to cooperate with medical assessments, it is worth making an extra effort ahead of time to find the best physician for the problem.

SEEKING OUT A QUALIFIED SPECIALIST

Most individuals have a primary care physician. A phone call or office visit to this doctor is a good place to start. Few, if any, primary care physicians will be comfortable making or confirming the diagnosis of FTD and managing the condition, since it is not common. Don't be surprised if your family doctor has not heard of it. Although often lacking the know-how to manage a patient with

FTD, they may know a specialist or cognitive disorders center that they have confidence in and work well with. This approach is most likely to enable you to gain access to experts experienced with FTD while maintaining a friendly relationship with the primary care physician.

If the affected individual does not have a primary care physician, most regions within the United States are associated with local branches of the Alzheimer's Association. These branches maintain listings of local physicians whom they recommend for the assessment of cognitive disorders. Local medical centers, hospitals, Web sites, and other referral centers may also be able to guide you to a capable physician.

Questions often arise regarding the type of medical specialist—neurologist, psychiatrist, or geriatrician—that is best qualified to care for the individual with frontotemporal dementia. In general, the neurologist has particular expertise in diagnostics. So if you are wondering whether an individual has FTD, Alzheimer's disease, or another condition, a neurologist may be the specialist to seek. The psychiatrist has particular expertise and interest in the management of behavioral symptoms. If there are behavioral problems that make the individual unsafe (e.g., agitated, destructive, aggressive, or violent behavior, or if the person is severely depressed or out of touch with reality) a psychiatrist may be of benefit. Psychiatrists are also helpful if the individual has had major side effects or a lack of response to medications that other doctors have prescribed for behavioral problems. However, some frontotemporal dementia patients are particularly reluctant to be evaluated by psychiatrists; in these cases, cognitive neurologists may be an option. Geriatricians are often recommended for older dementia patients with numerous other medical problems. However, the younger age of the average patient makes selection of a geriatrician less relevant for many.

Before committing yourself to one specialist, be aware that many exceptions to these general guidelines exist. Some neurologists are very adept at handling behavioral problems and some psychiatrists are good at arriving at the correct diagnosis. The most important quality in a specialist is that you are comfortable with the level of care that they can provide. It is more important to ensure that the physician has a clinical interest in frontotemporal dementia or degenerative diseases. You want the individual to be knowledgeable and skilled in handling the problems that arise, and interested in the patient.

Another issue to consider when selecting a physician is his willingness to discuss the patient in the patient's absence. With the exception of those with progressive aphasia, patients with frontotemporal dementia lack insight into their condition. It is sometimes difficult for caregivers to bring up the subject of cognitive loss when the patient is present in the examining room, for fear of embarrassing the patient or making him defensive. Doctors have different policies about discussing the patient when the patient is not present. Most physicians believe that information should be shared between the patient, caregiver, and doctor. Most do not wish to spend a long period of time away from the patient. The majority of doctors will discuss the situation briefly with family members if you indicate the need to do so. If there is a need to discuss the patient in his absence, ask about the doctor's policy on this ahead of time.

The presence of coordinated care or support services is also important. If diagnostic studies are needed, is there someone who can coordinate the visits to minimize the number of trips the patient needs to make to the hospital? If you need extra help or are unable to handle the individual in her current home setting, is there a social worker available? If the patient is falling or has problems with movements you may wish to identify a program with physical or occupational therapy. (See chapters 6, 11, and 12 for more information.) In general, physical therapists are effective when the person has trouble with falling, walking, or balance. A program with an occupational therapist should be targeted when upper extremity function is involved, including feeding, dressing, and cleaning. (For more information, see chapters 10 and 13.)

PREPARING TO VISIT THE DOCTOR

Before the appointment, you may wish to look up facts about FTD on Web sites or read about it so you are knowledgeable. It is wise to call the physician's office ahead of time to feel out the situation. You might want to ask if the doctor has other patients with this condition or if she has an interest in this area. Frontotemporal dementia patients don't always respond to treatments the same way as

Alzheimer's patients respond. This is because the underlying biology of the two diseases is different. So experience with Alzheimer's disease patients doesn't necessarily qualify a physician to manage patients with FTD.

When preparing for the visit, obtain copies of reports from blood work, EEGs, and from neuropsychologists. If specialized studies (X rays, MRI scans) have been done, bring copies of the studies, including copies of the actual X ray films. If possible, have all reports delivered in advance and call the office to be sure they have arrived. Do not assume that your doctor will have automatically forwarded copies of the old records.

THE DOCTOR'S EXAMINATION

During your initial appointment, you will want as many of your questions answered as possible. To get the most out of the appointment, prepare ahead for the encounter. At the time of the visit you should have a list of questions. If there are behavior problems or safety-related issues to discuss, be sure to bring them up. If the disease runs in the family, be sure to make the physician aware that this is a concern. Caregivers are also frequently anxious about prognostic information. This topic is often not discussed unless the caregiver brings it up.

In addition to taking a medical history and family history, the doctor will do a general physical examination, mental status examination, and general neurological examination. Do not have a patient with frontotemporal dementia go to the appointment without a caregiver or other informant. The physician will probably want to order some additional tests and may want to repeat some of the tests that have already been done. He may recommend genetic tests, cerebrospinal fluid (CSF) examination, or even brain biopsy.

In centers where there is a multidisciplinary approach to patient care, a nurse, physical therapist, neuropsychologist, or other healthcare professionals may be involved with the individual's care. In these cases, it is crucial to be sure there is good communication among the team members. Make sure that there is a system in place so that all the healthcare professionals on the team receive copies of all reports, and that the patient's primary care physician also receives copies.

FOLLOW-UP AFTER VISITING THE DOCTOR

After the appointment you may still want to know if this is the right doctor for you. Do you think the doctor is interested and knowledgeable about this problem? It is important that you get peace of mind from the physician and medical team. Were your questions answered? Was the problem treated seriously? Did he address safety issues? Were the X rays and blood work reviewed? Were blood work and imaging studies recommended to rule out conditions that mimic FTD? This is crucial. If the affected individual hasn't had a workup, and your doctor doesn't think a workup is warranted, you need another doctor.

Over time, a number of tests will be ordered and reordered. Changes in the studies can be as important diagnostically as the original results. As the caregiver, you should also keep copies of all diagnostic studies. If X rays or MRI scans are done, you should keep a copy of the films (not just the reports). These can be most easily obtained if requested at the time of the study. You are entitled to copies of these tests. Take these to the appointments. Also, when there is an upcoming physician appointment, call the office ahead of time to be sure that all new reports and X ray copies were received. It is surprising how often the results have not been received or reviewed.

Are you interested in clinical trials? In general, an institution with ongoing research programs may have active clinical expertise and clinical trials in your area of need. Many caregivers are interested in clinical trials for medications that help FTD. Unfortunately, because the disease is uncommon, most pharmaceutical companies are not funding large-scale trials for FTD. Additionally, since the diagnosis is much less common than Alzheimer's disease, some clinical trial sites are reluctant to engage in studies of FTD. Also, you will want a program where the physicians and staff are interested in patients outside of their candidacy as a clinical trial subject. If the site offers clinical trials, are the claims too good to be true? Specialty centers that make great promises about the effectiveness of medications for the type of symptoms FTD patients experience are often not legitimate. If you wish to select a center because it offers clinical trials, it is best to refer to your local Alzheimer's Association to be sure that the studies they offer are legitimate.

SUMMARY

Spending time to identify the right physician or program is often worthwhile when dealing with someone with frontotemporal dementia. Use your primary care physician and local resources to help guide you. FTD is much less common than Alzheimer's disease and few doctors are familiar with the issues that these patients experience. Make an effort to find a specialist with an interest in the area and get the most out of the first appointment by having results of prior testing organized and questions listed. As a bottom line, if you don't feel satisfied with the doctor or program, look for someone else.

CHAPTER 5

Therapeutic Interventions

Drug Treatments and Other Therapies

TIFFANY W. CHOW

GOALS OF THERAPY

The ideal treatment for chronic neurological illness would stop the process and restore normal function. At the present time, our understanding of neuroscience has not allowed us to recreate the complexity of thought and behavior in brains that have been damaged by dementia. Current research in therapies for dementia has two goals: interventions that can change the course of the illness, and treatment for isolated symptoms of the illness. Changing the course of the illness could mean reversing the losses, stopping any progression, or slowing the decline without being able to stop it altogether. Treatment for isolated symptoms relies upon the doctor's ability to untangle the crisis of dementia into a series of smaller, more familiar, and possibly easier problems to solve.

Interventions That Can Change the Course of Illness

Disease-modifying treatment for Alzheimer's disease is on the horizon. Due to important discoveries about what proteins build up abnormally in the brains of Alzheimer's patients, research has been able to focus on how to avoid production of the harmful protein clumps known more formally as plaques and tangles. Similar identification of abnormal proteins in FTD is a work in progress. We have some clues that tau, the protein that can serve as a building block for the tangles in AD, is also deranged in FTD, but we need more information on what specifically is wrong with tau in FTD patients. Until we know whether the problem is insufficient tau or not enough of the right type of tau, we can't start to administer a compound to right that wrong. Another way to change the course of FTD might be to stop the premature death of brain cells that occurs in frontal and temporal lobes. In this scenario, even if there were abnormal proteins in the vicinity, we could protect the brain cell (neuron) from being injured fatally. Future developments for AD patients that stop the death of neurons might also be useful for patients with FTD. In the meantime, drug treatment for AD patients that changes the amount of acetylcholine (a chemical messenger) in the brain does not change the course of FTD. There is currently no medication proven to halt the progression of FTD in any of its forms, which could be mainly behavioral, a primary progressive aphasia, or an illness very much like Lou Gehrig's disease (also known as amyotrophic lateral sclerosis or ALS).

Treatment for Isolated Symptoms of Frontotemporal Dementia

In the absence of an intervention that would stop the illness and return the patient to his baseline function, doctors consider FTD as a group of smaller problems that can be tackled individually. Approaching patient management with this perspective is referred to as symptomatic treatment. Medications or other nonpharmacologic interventions are then brought to bear on the case, based on their efficacy in treating each symptom, just one piece of the larger FTD puzzle. Table 1 at the end of the chapter lists the different types of symptoms that can occur in FTD patients. Not all patients will have all of these symptoms. In fact, most patients have only a few of these symptoms. One patient can have a few of these problems that evolve over time, showing new symptoms after the first ones fade away. The region of the brain that is most affected by illness usually determines which symptoms dominate the clinical picture. For instance, patients with more shrinkage (atrophy) of the right temporal lobe than other parts of the brain are more likely to have agitation, mania, and obsessive-compulsive behaviors throughout much of the illness than patients with atrophy focused on the brain's left side.

THE NATURE OF COGNITIVE CHANGES IN FRONTOTEMPORAL DEMENTIA

Behavioral neurologists divide the higher cognitive functions of the brain into seven domains: 1) attention, 2) frontal executive function, 3) language, 4) memory, 5) mood and personality, 6) spatial orientation, and 7) calculations. Each domain is not handled by only one location in the brain, but these labels allow us to group the numerous intellectual pursuits of the human brain. Frontotemporal dementia results in impairment of at least the first five of these cognitive domains. Alzheimer's disease, in comparison, affects all the domains except attention.

Attention refers to a person's ability to stay alert and focused on one particular activity. This cognitive domain must be up and running in order for a person to do well in the other cognitive domains. For example, if you can't pay close enough attention to what you're reading, you won't be able to remember it later on. Inattention is difficult to treat, but there may be some hope in following what clinicians use to treat Attention Deficit Disorder (ADD) in children, because these children have cognitive problems similar to those of FTD patients.

Frontal executive function is arguably the cognitive activity that makes us human. In its simplest sense, this cognitive domain allows a person to organize the world around him, to plan ahead, to build strategies, to monitor the outside environment in order to update the plan, and to prioritize the information he receives. When seen at a more complex level, this domain supports one's sense of humor, emotional activities, social skills, and creativity. Impairment of frontal executive function due to FTD results in devastating changes to personality and independent function. One drug has been tested to improve frontal executive dysfunction and will be discussed in the next section.

Language deficit is referred to as aphasia, which ranges from not being able to name things to misunderstanding what someone is saying despite being able to hear every word. Most types of aphasia that occur in FTD cannot be treated, but those who have difficulty getting the words out, nonfluent primary progressive aphasia, sometimes respond to oral medications that have been used more widely for patients with Parkinson's disease.

Memory loss can occur for different reasons. If it is related to inattention, then theoretically, regaining attentiveness will help; if the memory loss has been caused by damage to the machinery that lays down memories (temporal lobe structures), there is no current pharmacologic treatment available.

Mood and personality changes are discussed later in "Management of Behavioral Changes." Treating the cognitive disturbances of FTD symptomatically would target inattention, poor organizational and planning skills, aphasia, and memory loss.

PHARMACOLOGICAL TREATMENT FOR COGNITIVE CHANGES

Frontal Executive Dysfunction

It is possible that guanfacine (pronounced *gwon-fuh-seen*) could address frontal executive dysfunction in FTD. The American Food and Drug Adminstration (FDA) originally approved guanfacine as a blood pressure medication. Testing the drug on nonhuman primates indicated that this type of drug improved scores on frontal executive tests.[1] Later, eight- to sixteen-year-old children with ADD were treated with guanfacine and made significantly fewer errors on attention and frontal executive tests.[2] In another study, positive effects in subjects aged four to twenty were seen one month after starting the medication, and almost all of the subjects chose to continue the medication after the study was completed.[3] An open-label, prospective study at Rancho Los Amigos National Rehabilitation Center/USC Frontotemporal Dementia Clinic has tested the efficacy of guanfacine on eleven subjects with FTD.[4] The subjects took 0.5 mg of guanfacine daily for fourteen days. Dosage increased to 1 mg daily and stayed at this dose until day ninety—if blood pressure and pulse were stable at two weeks compared against baseline (premedication) vital signs. During the last month of the study, subjects took 1 mg twice daily. No one had significant changes in blood pressure during the study, which implies that the drug is safe to take, but the progression of dementia seemed to outweigh any benefit of the medication. While subjects improved a little on a few of the attention and frontal executive function tests, their scores declined on other tests over the four-month period or returned to baseline poor scores by the end of the study. Caregivers reported that two patients seemed more coherent during the study. Further investigation will determine whether the dose should be higher or if patients will only respond to the medication in the first few years of illness (the average duration of FTD in subjects was five years, which represented moderate to advanced stages) or if benefits of guanfacine were not measured adequately by the tests included in this study. Of note, there has been one case report of an FTD patient who improved with a similar drug called idazoxan.[5]

Treatment for Nonfluent Primary Progressive Aphasia

The primary progressive aphasias (PPA) run a relentless course, and only fluency of speech seems to have responded to pharmacotherapeutics in this sample of subjects. Comprehension of language has not been restored or stabilized with medications. Some investigators reported favorable responses to bromocriptine for aphasic subjects. M. L. Albert's case of mixed aphasia (problems with speech production and comprehension of spoken language) responded to 15 and 30 mg of bromocriptine per day; the subject complained of exacerbated vertigo at doses exceeding 30 mg.[6] Tanaka et al. improved naming performance in nonfluent aphasia due to stroke with doses of bromocriptine ranging from 2.5 to 7.5 mg per day.[7] It is not yet clear whether positive responses in subjects with stroke translate equally to those with nonfluent PPA.

Subjects with nonfluent PPA have felt some improvement in speech fluency, and caregivers report better alertness and motivation in response to amantadine. Other dopaminergic agents—bupropion, buspirone, and bromocriptine—have been tried but were either ineffective in my clinic or caused side effects before eliciting positive responses. Adverse effects of amantadine in five patients with NF-PPA have included: transient anxiety on 100 mg daily in one man; discoloration of skin on the legs (*livedo reticularis*) resolving after decrease to 100 mg daily in one man; exacerbation of gastroesophageal reflux disorder in one woman; dry mouth and constipation at 300 mg per day in one woman; and nightmares in another woman taking 300 mg per day.

MANAGEMENT OF BEHAVIORAL CHANGES

Table 1 at the end of this chapter lists the types of behavioral changes that we commonly face in my clinic. Comments below apply to observations drawn from thirty-five subjects followed at UCLA, then at Rancho Los Amigos National Rehabilitation Center/USC. The majority of subjects treated had one of the three types of PPA. Obsessive-compulsive behaviors and agitation were the most common behavioral disturbances among this group of subjects.

Depression, Anxiety, and Obsessive-Compulsive Behaviors

Alzheimer's disease patients typically have a deficiency of acetyl-choline. So far, FTD investigators have found more evidence for a deficiency of serotonin, another chemical messenger within the brain. There are many medications currently on the market to improve serotonin levels in the brain. They have been effective in treatment of mood disorders outside of the context of FTD, and they are advertised widely on television and in popular magazines. Since depression, anxiety, and obsessive-compulsive behaviors are also features of FTD, it makes sense to try the serotonergic medications, also known as SSRIs, or Selective Serotonin Reuptake Inhibitors.

Paroxetine was beneficial for 75 percent of subjects who took it, in that it decreased and eradicated repetitive, ritualistic behaviors. For example, a woman with FTD who compulsively stopped to rub or walk around certain trees while on daily walks with her dog was able to streamline the walks with less frequent stops. Patients with trichotillomania (constant tugging on hair or pulling it out) also responded to paroxetine. Bruxism (grinding the teeth) has been harder to extinguish with SSRIs. The drug is much more effective against repetitive behaviors than as an antidepressant or anxiolytic. Often, as subjects progressed, repetitive motor behaviors subsided, and in three subjects, paroxetine was successfully tapered to lower doses or discontinued completely.

Adverse effects with paroxetine included: stomach upset on 10 mg in one sixty-four-year-old man with semantic dementia, and exacerbation of anxiety and depression in a seventy-six-year-old woman with FTD. She also suffered decreased speech output at the starting dose of 10 mg per day. There was no complaint of headache or insomnia in twelve subjects, although these can be common side effects among patients treated with SSRIs.[8] Clomipramine, another type of SSRI, caused excessive sweating in a sixty-four-year-old man with semantic dementia when given for anxiety and obsessive-compulsive toileting behaviors. The same subject could not tolerate any SSRIs.

Clinicians frequently prescribe SSRIs for depression and anxiety.[9] Depressive symptoms did not respond, but anxiety was reduced with SSRIs. No clear antidepressant or anxiolytic effects were achieved with mirtazapine, bupropion, or buspirone.

Agitation and Psychosis

Agitation refers to yelling, combativeness, angry refusal of help, or physically violent acts. Psychosis refers to seeing or hearing things that aren't really there or believing a story that isn't true (e.g., "My deceased mother has been alive and well in the attic for the last two weeks.").

Agitation was most often treated with neuroleptic drugs. The least sedating and most effective neuroleptic medication was quetiapine. One subject developed moderate Parkinsonism on risperidone, which resolved after changing to quetiapine. Another subject made the same change to quetiapine after taking haloperidol, which caused moderate rigidity and blunted consciousness. Once on quetiapine, he was much more mobile, arrived at clinic ambulatory rather than by wheelchair, and was able to recognize close family members. Quetiapine replaced other typical and atypical neuroleptics when subjects developed Parkinsonism. Because of excessive sedation with olanzapine, another neuroleptic, two subjects were switched to quetiapine; one of these subjects had also experienced recurrence of seizures with olanzapine.

Patients with dementia are not immune to tardive dyskinesia, involuntary movements of the face or limbs, after receiving antipsychotic medication.[10] One woman with FTD in this series developed tardive dyskinesia six weeks after stopping haloperidol. Based on this study, neuroleptic use should be minimized and restricted to newer generation neuroleptics, such as quetiapine, olanzapine, and risperidone, to avoid exacerbating the Parkinsonism that commonly develops in later stages of FTD. Valproic acid has also been effective in addressing agitation in bid doses totaling 750 mg to 1125 mg per day.

A French team of clinicians has had success with trazodone for FTD patients. Trazodone at a dose of 150 mg split into three 50 mg doses per day then increased to 100 mg three times daily reduced agitation, irritability, anxiety, and delusions in fourteen subjects observed over a six-week period.[11] The drug's most common side effect is drowsiness, but the subjects in this study did not complain of this problem.

Benzodiazepines (e.g., lorazepam or diazepam) are frequently used to calm or sedate people in a variety of circumstances, but their use in patients with dementia is controversial. Most FTD investigators find that benzodiazepines enhance confusion and have a prolonged half-life in FTD patients and thus are better avoided.

Sexual disinhibition in FTD can be very distressing to family members and increases risk of harm to the patient. Premarin at a dose of .625 mg daily has ended inappropriate sexual advances from two men; one had NF-PPA, the other semantic dementia. SSRIs commonly create sexual dysfunction among young patients with depression or anxiety, and this adverse effect for them may be a desirable side effect in a patient with FTD and sexual disinhibition.

Insomnia Is Hard to Treat

Only three of the thirty-five subjects had insomnia requiring sedatives in addition to an SSRI or valproic acid. A seventy-eight-year-old woman with Parkinsonian FTD responded to trazodone, 25 to 50 mg at bedtime. A fifty-year-old woman became oversedated with 50 mg of trazodone. A sixty-nine-year-old man with semantic dementia was reported by his caregivers to sleep only two hours in twenty-four for over six months. Trazodone was not increased beyond 50 mg PO qHS (at bedtime, orally), because the starting dose increased agitation. Fortunately, the insomnia has resolved in this subject despite his resistance to multiple treatments, and insomnia is not a major complaint for other subjects at this clinic.

MOTOR CHANGES

Signs of Parkinson's Disease

As FTD progresses, many patients experience a slowing (bradykinesia) and rigidity to their movements, which may be accompanied by loss of balance and frequent falls because they cannot right themselves quickly enough. I have observed results with two medications for this problem: carbidopa/levodopa and amantadine. One subject had relief of bradykinesia and rigidity with 25 mg carbidopa/100 mg levodopa twice daily. Another subject with both nonfluent PPA and Parkinsonism had improvement in speech and bradykinesia with a low dose of carbidopa/levodopa; development of psychosis and vivid dreams prohibited higher dosing. Unfortunately, this adverse effect is the downside of anti-Parkinsonian medications. Amantadine improved alertness and increased speech fluency transiently (i.e., for a few months).

Anti-ALS Medication Has Not Been Beneficial for Patients with Motor Weakness

Although there are links between ALS and FTD, two syndromes featuring rapidly progressive muscle weakness and wasting,[12] the drug approved by the FDA for treatment of ALS, riluzole, did not prevent rapid deterioration in subjects seen at my clinic with this type of FTD. There is no evidence to support use of riluzole in patients with FTD without the muscle weakness and wasting.

NONPHARMACOLOGIC INTERVENTIONS

Acupuncture and Herbal Medicine

The theory behind this practice overlaps with the neurological idea of cognitive domains stated previously. The acupuncturist and herbalist do not separate bodily or constitutional components from cognitive domains, however. Therefore, the heart system must be treated in order to address emotional function; the spleen or digestive organs are related to mental processing; kidney to memory; liver to nerves in the limbs; and lung to mental and physical flexibility.

Two patients with FTD were referred to an acupuncturist who is also well versed in herbal medicine and massage therapy. Although both patients carry the same general diagnosis of FTD, their key symptoms were different and warranted very different diagnoses within the Eastern medicine model. The first woman had the NF-PPA type of presentation, along with complaints of shooting pains in the back of her neck and top of her head. The acupuncturist said her condition represented "Stagnation of Heart" in a Fire Body Type. She was treated with combinations of acupuncture, electrical stimulation, and moxibustion* at some needling sites, and massage therapy weekly over a six-week period. Targets for treatment were pericardium, urinary bladder, gall bladder, and governing vessel channels. The last three channels are also manipulated when acupuncturists are treating patients with epilepsy, memory loss, Bell's palsy (facial paralysis), and unconsciousness. During the treatment period, our patient showed reopening of the pericardium (heart) channels, which manifested physically as coughing up phlegm. This patient was seen in the clinic during the six-week period and found to be much less agitated and painfree. The acupuncturist reported that she became more animated and alert, showing an understanding of the context of the office visits and increased cooperation. The patient's move out of the country to be cared for by her extended family interrupted her treatment. Ordinarily, someone like her who had responded quickly (within the first few treatments) would be continued up to eight to twelve weeks.

The other patient was a woman with muscle slowing and rigidity, as well as bruxism (grinding the teeth) and drooling as predominant features of FTD. Her diagnosis for acupuncture and herbal medical treatment was "Spleen Chi Deficiency" in an Earth Body Type. The drooling responded well to combinations of acupuncture, electrical stimulation, and moxibustion at some needling sites, massage therapy, and a lemon extract. This patient experienced weekly treatment for a month, but traveling from her home to the acupuncture clinic was too difficult due to her problems with mobility. A deficiency takes longer to treat than a blockage (see first patient

---

*A technique to enhance the efficacy of a needling procedure, where a flammable substance is added to the exposed end of the needle.

described), and the general rule of thumb is that the treatment for deficiency may take one month per year of underlying illness.[13]

I have not been trained in Eastern medicine and have made an attempt here to paraphrase what my consulting friend explained to me. The important themes are: (1) this type of medicine allows a completely different perspective on the causes of the illness and approaches to correct its symptoms and (2) it takes time to see efficacy of the treatment, especially if the illness has been long-standing prior to evaluation. Interested readers can get information from the book *The Web That Has No Weaver: Understanding Chinese Medicine,* 2d ed., by Ted Kaptchuk (Lincolnwood, Ill.: Contemporary Books, 2000) or *Between Heaven and Earth: A Guide to Chinese Medicine* by Harriet Beinfield and Efrem Korngold (New York: Ballantine, 1992), for more details.

Behavioral Interventions

Techniques used by psychologists to help patients change their behaviors are called behavior modifications. These can be very effective for training people to kick habits such as smoking, nailbiting, tics, and obsessive-compulsive behaviors, or even to address phobias. Behavior modification cannot succeed without a patient's ability to monitor himself for the undesired behavior and without the patient's wish to end the behavior. In the case of a patient with FTD, then, behavioral modification will only work earlier in the course of illness, when the patient can still recognize problem behaviors as undesirable and when he can be trained to do something new.

Lough describes modest success providing behavioral modification therapy to a fifty-seven-year-old man with marked behavioral changes due to FTD.[14] The case is a little unusual in that the patient had first shown symptoms more than a decade prior to receiving treatment, yet he could still score perfectly on a brief mental status examination. This retained cognitive ability probably allowed him to benefit from the treatment, although other patients with similar length of illness and severity of behavioral problems might not be able to benefit from the therapy. Dr. Lough's patient had apathy, disinhibition, a preference for sweets, inappropriate giggling, grandiose and paranoid delusions, irritability, obsessive-compulsive behaviors, and tendency to wander. The therapists were able to train the patient not to shove automobiles compulsively by replacing that behavior with visual inspection of cars, and special signs were posted at doorways to prevent the patient from wandering off the hospital ward. Instead of saying, STOP, the signs urged the patient to TURN AROUND. Although only two of the patient's behaviors could be targeted, addressing those significantly improved the patient's safety, tolerability to others, and quality of life.

Some patients with depression or anxiety may benefit from one-on-one psychotherapy, but this depends upon their communication skills. Some may argue that the patient feels better while in session but quickly forgets the intervention at home. Whether this is at least helpful in a transient sense is a philosophical issue. Certainly caregivers have benefited from counseling and caregiver support group interactions, and this indirectly improves the patient's quality of life.

FURTHER COMMENTS

Despite lack of a cholinergic deficit in subjects with FTD, most clinicians prescribe donepezil to patients before referring them to the FTD clinic. It is not clear whether this is due to misdiagnosis as an atypical presentation of AD or an attempt to try a cognitive-enhancing agent in the absence of disease-modifying medications for FTD, but donepezil has not benefited subjects who meet clinical diagnostic criteria for FTD.

Need for Clinical Drug Trials

As a collection of anecdotal observations, the recommendations for behavioral management with medications presented here clearly have limited applicability to other FTD patients. This was not a blinded, controlled study of medication efficacy. Frequency of prescribed medications in this review was biased by prior response to medications. If all medications were prescribed to all subjects with the target symptoms in a formal experiment, perhaps more subjects would have responded. The impact of several medications given simultaneously to a patient is not yet clear. Conclusions from this review must be understood in this context, and demands from treating physicians should be tempered to using these recommendations as a springboard for discussion of medication decision making.

The best way to prove a given medication's efficacy for treating a specific patient population is to carry out formal clinical drug trials that have been reviewed by an institutional Human Subjects Protection Committee. The guanfacine study described in this chapter was approved by a Human Subjects Protection Committee, but all participants received medication, as opposed to half taking placebo and half taking the medication. Without information on patients who weren't taking guanfacine, one cannot tell whether the drug at least slowed the progression of illness over the four-month period.

Formal clinical drug trials are expensive and time-consuming. Devoting more resources to FTD research at local and federal levels will enable investigators to carry out meaningful studies. Any new medications to be approved for FTD would require review by the FDA, the official government agency responsible for ensuring that our drug supply is safe and effective. At the very beginning, a pharmaceutical company initiates laboratory testing to estimate the effectiveness and safety of a proposed drug product. This proceeds into testing on animals. The company then communicates its intentions to the FDA, because it will start testing the new drug on humans. The process of dialogue with the FDA can be long, in addition to the time it takes to conduct the research itself. The FDA's Center for Drug Evaluation and Research (CDER) evaluates the results of laboratory and animal testing prior to approving testing in humans.

Three phases of trials are conducted on human subjects before the drug can be approved for public use with a doctor's prescription. Phase I clinical trials require a small number (twenty to eighty) of healthy people who don't necessarily share the same characteristics as the target patient group. For example, subjects in a Phase I clinical trial for a drug eventually to be used for FTD may be college-aged volunteers and completely without cognitive impairment. This phase of testing is meant to establish drug chemistry, safety, adverse reactions, and proper dosage in humans. Phase II clinical trials are similar to Phase I trials except the drug is given to a larger (one hundred to three hundred) group of participants, and these subjects would actually have FTD. This phase of testing also helps determine the frequency of short-term side effects and risks associated with the drug when used in the target population. Phase III trials recruit a larger sample (one thousand to three thousand) to monitor for reactions to the drug and the drug's effectiveness when compared to existing treatments.

Data from these studies allow assessment of the overall benefit-risk relationship of the drug and ability to apply the results to the larger population of patients. Satisfactory completion of the three types of trials with demonstration of clear benefit over risk of side effects can lead to FDA approval of the drug. The following Web sites provide further information on this subject: www.fda.gov/cder/ and www.coreynahman.com/FDA_Page.html.

Just because a drug is being used in Europe does not mean it automatically qualifies for FDA approval. The pharmaceutical company may not have to repeat the European clinical trials already performed to meet European standards, but it must present those results to the FDA and show proper evidence for the three types of clinical trials before it is approvable in this country. When prescribing a medication for FTD patients that has already gained FDA approval for another disease, the clinician should clearly inform the patient and family that this is an off-label use of the drug. For example, amantadine has FDA approval for use as an antiviral and an anti-Parkinson's disease agent, and it has adequately proven safety for use in humans, but it may benefit patients with NF-PPA (see earlier discussion). Before prescribing the amantadine, though, the clinician should explain the experimental nature of this particular prescription. At an academic clinic like the one at USC, the patient signs an informed consent so that no one is misled about the expectations for treatment with the drug.

SUMMARY

Based on the experiences at my clinics, the most effective SSRI was paroxetine, but this was more useful for repetitive, ritualistic behaviors than either depression or anxiety. Amantadine was effective for increasing fluency and attention in subjects with NF–PPA but not semantic dementia. Quetiapine and valproic acid are well-tolerated antipsychotics and may be useful to control extremely disruptive behaviors that break through a high dose of SSRI. Trazodone also should be considered for treatment of agitation. Parkinsonism is exacerbated by haloperidol. There is no clear recommendation for pharmacologic antidepressant therapy, although depressive symptoms are common in patients with FTD. Riluzole and donepezil have not shown positive effects in subjects with unequivocal diagnosis of a frontotemporal dementia.

Multicenter, double-blind, placebo-controlled studies of each psychotropic medication would yield the most scientifically reliable data on medications useful for the frontotemporal dementias. Collaborations between centers which can agree on subgroup classifications of frontotemporal dementias may be able to create studies with sufficient power.

TABLE 1. Targets for Symptomatic Treatment

Cognitive Changes
> Inattention
> Poor concentration
> Poor planning
> Perseveration (uncontrollable repetition)
> Nonfluent aphasia

Behavioral Changes
> Depression
> Anxiety
> Agitation
> Obsessive-compulsive behaviors
> Psychosis
> Insomnia
> Sexual disinhibition

Changes in Bodily Movement
> Parkinsonism
> Muscle weakness and wasting (as in amyotrophic lateral sclerosis)

NOTES

1. A. F. Arnsten and P. S. Goldman-Rakic, "Alpha 2-adrenergic mechanisms in prefrontal cortex associated with cognitive decline in aged nonhuman primates," *Science* 230 (1985): 1273–76; J. X. Cai et al., "Reserpine impairs spatial working memory performance in monkeys: reversal by the

alpha-2 adrenergic agonist clonidine," *Brain Research* 614 (1993): 191–96; A. F. Arnsten, J. X. Cai, and P. S. Goldman-Rakic, "The alpha-2 adrenergic agonist guanfacine improves memory in aged monkeys without sedative or hypotensive side effects: Evidence for alpha-2 receptor subtypes," *Journal of Neuroscience* 8 (1988): 4287–98; A. F. Arnsten and F. M. Leslie, "Behavioral and receptor binding analysis of the alpha-2 adrenergic agonist, 5-bromo-6 [2-imidazoline-2-yl amino] quinoxaline (UK-14304): Evidence for cognitive enhancement at an alpha-2 adrenoceptor subtype," *Neuropharmacology* 30 (1991): 1279–89; P. Rama et al., "Medetomidine, atipamezole, and guanfacine in delayed response performance of aged monkeys," *Pharmacology, Biochemistry, and Behavior* 55 (1996): 415–22; J. S. Franowicz and A. F. Arnsten, "The alpha-2a noradrenergic agonist, guanfacine, improves delayed response performance in young adult rhesus monkeys," *Psychopharmacology* 136 (1998): 8–14.

2. P. B. Chappell et al., "Guanfacine treatment of comorbid attention-deficit hyperactivity disorder and Tourette's syndrome: Preliminary clinical experience," *Journal of the American Academy of Child and Adolescent Psychiatry* 34 (1995): 1140–46; P. Jakala et al., "Guanfacine, but not clonidine, improves planning and working memory performance in humans," *Neuropsychopharmacology* 20 (1999): 460–70; P. Jakala et al., " Guanfacine and clonidine, alpha-2 agonists, improve paired associates learning, but not delayed matching to sample, in humans," *Neuropsychopharmacology* 20 (1999): 119–30.

3. R. D. Hunt, A. F. Arnsten, and M. D. Asbell, "An open trial of guanfacine in the treatment of attention-deficit hyperactivity disorder," *Journal of the American Academy of Child and Adolescent Psychiatry* 34 (1995): 50–54.

4. T. W. Chow, "Open label trial of guanfacine in frontotemporal dementia," *American Journal of Alzheimer's Disease and Other Dementias* 17, no. 5 (2002): 267–72.

5. B. J. Sahakian, J. J. Coull, and J. R. Hodges, "Selective enhancement of executive function by idazoxan in a patient with dementia of the frontal lobe type," *Journal of Neurology, Neurosurgery & Psychiatry* 57 (1994): 120–21.

6. M. L. Albert et al., "Pharmacotherapy for aphasia," *Neurology* 38 (1988): 877–79.

7. Y. Tanaka et al., "Dopamine agonist improves speech output in non-fluent aphasia," *Neurology* 54 (2000): A102.

8. G. Chouinard et al., "A Canadian multicenter, double-blind study of paroxetine and fluoxetine in major depressive disorder," *Journal of Affective Disorders* 54 (1999): 39–48.

9. R. Swartz et al., "Behavioral phenomenology in Alzheimer's disease, frontotemporal dementia, and late-life depression: A retrospective analysis," *Journal of Geriatric Psychiatry and Neurology* 10 (1997): 67–74.

10. T. M. Magnuson et al., "Medication-induced dystonias in nine patients with dementia," *Journal of Neuropsychiatry and Clinical Neurosciences* 12 (2000): 219–25.

11. F. Lebert and F. Pasquier, "Trazodone in the treatment of behaviour in frontotemporal dementia," [letter to the editor], *Human Psychopharmacology* 14 (1999): 279–81.

12. Y. Mitsuyama, "Presenile dementia with motor neuron disease," *Dementia* 4 (1993): 137–42; W. M. Hooten and C. G. Lyketsos, "Frontotemporal dementia: a clinicopathological review of four postmortem studies," *Journal of Neuropsychiatry and Clinical Neurosciences* 8 (1996): 10–19; D. Neary et al., "Frontotemporal lobar degeneration: A consensus on clinical diagnostic criteria," *Neurology* 51 (1998): 1546–54.

13. Daniel Bagdadi, L. Ac., personal communication, 22 January 2002.

14. S. Lough and J. R. Hodges, "Measuring and modifying abnormal social cognition in frontal variant frontotemporal dementia," *Journal of Psychosomatic Research* 53 (2002): 639–43.

CHAPTER 6

Rehabilitation Interventions:
Uses and Benefits of Speech, Occupational, and Physical Therapies

KEITH M. ROBINSON

THE IDEA BEHIND REHABILITATION

Rehabilitation is a holistic, comprehensive treatment approach that incorporates the physical, cognitive, behavioral, emotional, and social dimensions of care. It operates as a physician-directed team effort that is multidisciplinary in membership and interdisciplinary in process. Rehabilitation treatments focus on everyday life functions that need to be restored or modified for an individual to maintain an optimal level of control within his meaningful environment. For the individual with a dementia, the goal of rehabilitation is to maintain the highest level of empowerment that is realistically and safely possible through restorative and preventative/maintenance treatments performed collaboratively by therapists, the individual, and her caregivers.

Restorative treatments are those that require specialized interventions by therapists to re-achieve a previously established functional level that has become compromised by acute illness and/or by dementia. For example, the recovery from an aspiration pneumonia in an individual with a frontotemporal dementia inevitably will require a period of inactivity. The physiologic impact of this event will cause a loss of ability to walk, care for oneself, and interact with others.

Preventative/maintenance treatments are those that are performed by the individual autonomously or with the supervision and assistance of caregivers, often as the product of restorative treatments, to maintain the highest level of functioning possible for the individual. Preventative/maintenance treatments are viewed as at least as important as restorative treatments because they define, in part, the daily routines of the individual.

Rehabilitation treatments do not separate the individual from her caregivers and from the environment in which she lives. Rehabilitation defines the caregivers broadly to include family members, friends, neighbors, fellow church community members, volunteers, and skilled/semiskilled personnel (e.g., home health aides, homemakers), as those who supervise or assist the individual with a dementia in his community-based or institutional place of residence. Rehabilitation views the social support system as the interpersonal environment, and the place of residence as the physical environment.

Therapeutic interventions are directed toward the individual and these environments concurrently. For example, in those individuals who have progressed in their dementia to the point where learning is finite, rehabilitation directs treatments toward these environments to educate caregivers in rational care of the individual (e.g., cueing someone with aspiration risk to tuck her chin during swallowing), and to create a physically safe environment to reduce risks of physical injury to an individual or caregiver (e.g., training the spouse of someone who has excessive involuntary movement how to properly move the person.)

Rehabilitation emphasizes the mundane in everyday life, that is, those activities in which everyone must participate, (e.g., eat, toilet) to negotiate through the day. When considering dementia, control of one's rituals in everyday life is dynamically defined by how far an individual has progressed in her disease trajectory. Loss of function is inevitable. Redefining optimal control as loss occurs is operationalized by rehabilitation strategies. Optimal control, regardless of functional status, can invoke a less negative perception of one's declining situation and a higher sense of quality of life.

Despite loss, particularly of cognitive functions, learning new or alternative ways of participating in everyday life rituals is possible for the individual with FTD, particularly in the early and middle stages of the disease. As remembering names, places, and events becomes difficult and less important, remembering procedures can remain relatively spared. The former type of conscious learning known as declarative or explicit—or the "learning what" memory system—becomes impaired in dementia. The latter type of unconscious learning known as procedural or implicit—or the "learning how" memory system—can remain relatively available for learning other methods to negotiate safely through everyday life, such as learning to sequence a walker to ambulate.

Rehabilitation views inactivity as harmful to health and well-being. There are well-documented negative anatomic, physiological and psychological effects of inactivity, summarized in table 1 on pages 109–10. Bed rest, although sometimes a necessary treatment to recover from an acute episode of illness, has negative side effects that can be as disastrous as the side effects of medications. Much of the effort of rehabilitation is directed toward reversing and minimizing these negative effects.

THE ESSENTIAL TOOLS OF REHABILITATION

Functional assessment is the basic method of clinical evaluation to define rehabilitation treatments and to determine the utility or outcome from treatments. The multidisciplinary team operationalizes treatment approaches.

Functional Assessment

Rehabilitation defines function at the level of individual performance in relation to other people who are caregivers within a meaningful environment where one lives. Function in these terms does not view the individual as the deconstructed collection of cells, neurotransmitters, and organ systems that comprises his anatomic and physiologic protoplasm, but rather as how this protoplasm performs basic survival skills to negotiate through everyday life and what is the burden of care on others to perform these skills successfully. Functional assessment observes and measures performance in three broad areas of living: communication, self-care, and mobility. Each of these three areas can be categorized into those that are necessary to survive within one's home or place of residence, and those that are necessary to survive in the larger community. These functional survival skills are summarized in table 2 on p. 111.

The Rehabilitation Team

The core rehabilitation team includes a rehabilitation medical specialist, that is, a physiatrist, and three nonmedical specialists: speech therapist, physical therapist, and occupational therapist. Each of these specialists traditionally has been considered an expert in treating deficits in each of the three broad areas of functioning: speech therapists treat communication deficits; occupational therapists treat self-care deficits; and physical therapists treat mobility deficits. Over time, their respective areas of expertise have evolved to include treating functional deficits that require overlapping and complementary approaches. For example, as speech therapists assess and treat swallowing deficits, occupational therapists concurrently assess and treat fine motor strategies that control eating/feeding. These therapy disciplines are more thoroughly defined and discussed in chapters 10 through 14.

The rehabilitation team also includes a larger array of nonmedical specialists who operationalize clinical assessments and treatment interventions collaboratively, either based on a prescription or referral from a physician (e.g., neurologist, primary care doctor, physiatrist), or by cross-referral from another nonmedical member of the team. Table 3 on pages 112–14 summarizes the division of labor among the rehabilitation specialists. Rehabilitation includes the individual's caregivers as an essential component of the team, because they continue to operationalize strategies during preventative/maintenance interventions learned during restorative and skilled treatments.

While any physician can prescribe rehabilitation treatments, the physiatrist understands best the skills of the various team members, and in doing so, often functions as the gatekeeper of rehabilitation services. The physiatrist plays a major role in defining precautions for rehabilitation interventions for therapists, particularly exercise, which can be performed even by severely debilitated individuals. The physiatrist, by forming a partnership with the primary care physician or neurologist, manages the rehabilitation aspects of treatment in coordination with the medical management. The physiatrist will manage the following:

1. Prescribe, monitor, and revise rehabilitation services.
2. Decide which nonmedical specialists are appropriate to intervene at specific points in time.

3. Reinforce the execution of preventative/maintenance treatments by the social support system.
4. Decide on the best site for rehabilitation services to occur (inpatient, outpatient, home).
5. Prescribe durable medical equipment (DME) such as walkers, wheelchairs, and commodes.

SPECIFIC TREATMENT APPROACHES

Minimizing Deconditioning

Deconditioning is a syndrome that is comprised of the reversible and preventable negative anatomic and physiologic effects of bed rest, inactivity, and sedentary lifestyles. It affects multiple organ systems and is cumulative, superimposing the effects of the underlying neurodegenerative process and its complications that sometime necessitate immobilization. There are commonsensical interventions that therapists can teach caregivers to minimize its effects. Some of these treatments include: daily muscle and joint range-of-motion to minimize the effects of spasticity in forming soft-tissue contractures, regular walking programs and upper limb repetitive activities to prevent loss of stamina and endurance, and the use of wheelchair cushions and mattresses made of specialized materials to decompress bony weight-bearing sites to prevent pressure sores. They are summarized in table 1 on pages 109–10.

Contractures occur when joints and their associated soft tissues (tendons, ligaments, muscles) are immobilized for prolonged periods of time. They worsen as the period of immobility lengthens. What occurs is a progressive shortening and remolding of musculoskeletal tissues into positions that can interfere with performing basic survival skills (e.g., mobilizing the shoulder for eating, lifting up the foot and ankle for walking, cleaning skin folds of the armpit, the fingers and wrists, and between the legs.) Contractures can be minimized with range-of-motion and gentle muscle flexibility programs taught by physical and occupational therapists.

Loss of muscle strength and loss of the endurance of muscles to perform repetitive activities without excessive fatigue can start to occur within a few days of bed rest, and worsen as the period of immobilization lengthens. Immobilization can augment aging-related bone demineralization (osteoporosis), increasing the risk of a bone fracture during minor trauma. Muscle weakness and loss of muscle endurance, and osteoporosis can be minimized with conservative strengthening and muscle endurance exercises, such as bedside strengthening; sustained sitting at the bedside or upright in a supportive chair; prewalking activities such as repetitive sitting to standing, weight shifting during sustained standing and walking in place; gait training with an assistive device such as a walker. The physical therapist usually takes the lead in teaching the individual and caregivers these mobility skills.

Important risk factors for pressure sores in individuals with FTD include involuntary movement disorders such as spasticity and rigidity that disallow smooth motor control, incontinence with frequent moistening of the skin, poor nutrition, poor initiation, and sensory deficits at weight-bearing sites over bony prominences such as the shoulder blades and the buttocks. Prevention of pressure sores is a multidisciplinary effort including: bed mobility and transfer training to avoid shearing or friction during movement (physical therapy), repositioning schedules during sustained sitting and when in bed (physical therapy, occupational therapy, and wound specialist nurses in hospital or home care), specialized cushions and mattresses to decompress weight-bearing sites (physical therapy and nursing), and specialized foot and ankle bracing to unload the heels when in bed such as a multipodis boots (physical therapy, nursing, and orthotics).

The effects of immobilization on the heart, lungs, and blood vessels include an increase in resting heart rate, an abrupt increase in heart rate with minimal activity, and a decrease in cardiac reserve to perform sustained everyday life activities, resulting in easy fatiguabilty. The output of blood from the heart during each contraction to supply vital organs decreases. The integrity of the muscles inside of veins and arteries becomes compromised; thus, resting blood pressure becomes lower and drops with changes in position from lying to sitting to standing, resulting in dizziness and passing out (orthostatic hypotension). The efficiency of breathing becomes compromised because of loss of strength of the ventilatory muscles and collapse of the more dependent segments of the lung, resulting in inconsistent and irregular air exchange from the airways into the blood stream. The protective cough reflex weakens; clearance of secretions becomes less effective, increasing the risk of food, mucous, and gastric contents to enter the lungs (aspiration). Vascular blood flow in the leg veins slows down, predisposing the individual to blood clot formation in the deeper large veins (deep venous thrombosis). If these clots break into small pieces, they can travel to the lungs and interfere with blood flow and air exchange. This is life threatening and known as a pulmonary embolism. Both a deep venous thrombosis and a pulmonary embolism require treatment with a blood thinner such as Coumadin, which has its own risk of easier bleeding with minor trauma, particularly in people who fall frequently. These cardiovascular and pulmonary consequences of inactivity can be minimized with several therapeutic interventions: graduated sitting, standing, and walking programs (physical therapy); no/low resistance, high repetition strengthening exercises such as ankle pumps (physical therapy); ventilatory muscle training; and swallowing assessment and individualized strategies such as changing food consistencies and specific head and neck positions to prevent aspiration (speech therapy).

Cognitive Remediation of Intellectual Deficits

Dementia is defined by progressive cognitive and intellectual losses. Neuroscientific investigation has made promising headway into understanding the underlying cellular and neurochemical mechanisms that underpin cognitive functions. Treatment of the cognitive deficits that occur with dementias and other brain disorders is limited by what we know about fundamental brain mechanisms and how these have been applied to clinical diagnosis. A more sophisticated appreciation of cognition, intelligence, and learning is evolving. New models of cognition, intelligence, and learning are being developed and tested through scientific pursuit in a variety of brain disorders. The models that have been developed from studying other diagnoses, such as head injury, multiple sclerosis, and stroke, can be applied to treating dementia, particularly in the early and middle stages of the disease trajectory. With these thoughts in mind, several principles can be articulated about rehabilitation of cognitive and intellectual deficits, that is, cognitive remediation:

1. A hierarchy of cognitive functions is assumed. Attentional functions and short term memory can be viewed as infrastructure that support more complex cognitive processes. Treating attention and short-term memory deficits with a combination of neuromodulating medications and behaviorally based treatments may enhance performance of more complex cognitive functions. A fundamental approach used to treat behavioral impairments in cognitive infrastructure includes repetition and guided forced usage. However, in treating individuals with dementia, practice will not make perfect, but it may improve function and safety by enhancing attentional systems.

2. Despite common deficits that define dementia, every individual with dementia has her own idiosyncratic profile of intellectual strengths and deficits. Detailed behavioral, neurological, and neuropsychological assessment is the best approach to define an individual's profile of cognitive strengths and weaknesses. This profile then can be translated by various members of the rehabilitation team (neuropsychologist, speech therapist, occupational therapist) into behaviorally based cognitive remediation strategies that are task and goal specific.

3. Learning theory has distinguished the two different systems of learning mentioned above: the conscious/explicit/declarative/ "learning what" system, and the unconscious/implicit/ procedural "learning how" system. The former system has a more specific localization of neural networks in the brain, connecting the medial temporal lobes with specific areas of the thalamus, the base of the frontal lobes, and the amygdala. The medial temporal lobes sustain particular damage in dementia with deficits in its associated "learning what" system. The latter "learning how" system has a more diffuse representation in the brain and is certainly subject to damage in dementia, yet theoretically may be relatively spared as a learning system until the later stages of disease. Much of what underpins rehabilitation treatments, including cognitive remediation, is dependent on the "learning how" system in that what occurs is teaching cognitive and motor skills and procedures that are task and goal specific, as well as behav-

iorally based, and that either accommodate or compensate for neurological deficits.

4. Cognitive remediation involves two fundamental approaches: utilizing cognitive strengths to bypass cognitive weaknesses, and replacing "lost" information and procedures with external aids. Common examples of a bypass strategy is the procedural motor learning that occurs when a person is required to sequence a walker to walk safely and to reduce falling risk in physical therapy. Another example is when a person is taught to use chin tuck and double swallow maneuvers in speech therapy to minimize aspiration risk during eating. A common example of the use of external aids is procedurally learning the use of daily planners and memory logs to cue the retrieval of critical information necessary for negotiating through everyday life, such as types and times of medication usage, appointments, and safe meal preparation procedures.

5. Cognitive remediation often links the use of physician-prescribed neuromodulating medications, with behaviorally based treatments that are encompassed by procedural learning, and with structured and nonpunitive behavioral management. It is of fundamental importance that the treating rehabilitation team be made aware when such medications are initiated, modified, and discontinued, so that the therapists can closely observe with caregivers any beneficial/detrimental effects of medication interventions by using behavior trackers that monitor precipitants, instances, and quality of targeted behaviors.

Procedural learning in the context of rehabilitation is task and goal specific. More complex tasks are deconstructed into a logical sequence of steps that are reconstructed during treatment. The learning that occurs tends to become hyperspecific for the targeted task; for example, learning the use of a remote control device to control cable television channels should not presume that this learning will generalize to apply to successful use of a cell phone. See chapter 5 for a more in-depth discussion of neuromodulating medications.

Treatment of Difficult or Unruly Behaviors

While progressive cognitive deficits define the presence of a dementia, they are often associated with difficult or problematic behaviors. When they occur, they can be unsafe for the individual and her caregivers, and can interfere with meaningful participation in therapies. Some of these behaviors include: poor initiation, easy distractibility, agitation, wandering, disinhibition, anger, aggression, poor insight or self monitoring of one's abilities and inabilities, poor communication skills, perseveration or "getting stuck" in the middle of an activity, emotional lability, and obsessiveness-compulsivity. Often, they require neuromodulating agents to control (see chapter 5). Knowledge of some basic principles of behavioral management that are incorporated into rehabilitation treatments can assist caregivers in exercising more control in creating a safe interpersonal environment. These include:

1. The environment in which the individual with dementia lives should be structured, consistent, and have minimally distracting influences. This will at least encourage appropriate activity participation to support a normal sleep-wake cycle.
2. Every effort should be made to ensure that the individual's hearing and vision are optimized since they control the primary entry of sensory information from the environment into the brain.
3. Many disturbing behaviors have specific precipitators that can be identified, then modified or eliminated. When a pattern cannot be realized, fatigue from environmental overload should be entertained as an explanation, and "down time" and short naps should be included in the structured daily schedule.
4. Desirable and adaptive behaviors should be rewarded with positive feedback. Undesirable behaviors should be responded to as neutrally as is safely possible. Positive feedback seems an easier and more enjoyable response and usually involves a simple positive emotional message such as a smile, verbal encouragement, or touch. Neutral responses to problematic behaviors seem counterintuitive; however, negative feedback simply reinforces a target behavior by serving it with more attention. Neutral responses in these situations

can be difficult to adopt by family members intimately involved with the individual with dementia because this requires modifying longstanding patterns of behavioral responses that have fueled close relationships. Furthermore, eliciting a neutral response is not always safe in situations in which an individual is being injurious to self and others. The use of "time out" or removing the individual from an environment may be useful in this situation.

Treatment of Involuntary Movement Disorders: Rigidity and Spasticity

Rigidity and spasticity are two involuntary movement disorders seen in individuals with dementia. In many patients they can be difficult to distinguish, particularly in the middle and later stages of disease. Rigidity is one of several Parkinsonian signs that disallows smooth and fluid motor control during daily life activities. The individual subjectively experiences stiffness, and expends more energy to perform basic survival skills such as eating and walking, resulting in easy fatiguability. It can also increase falling risk.

Spasticity can be distinguished from rigidity by an involuntary resistance to an external stretch to a specific muscle group that is "velocity dependent." The more rapidly that one provides an external stretch, the more resistance by the muscle is observed. When there is demonstrated functional interference, spasticity should be treated with antispasticity medications (e.g., dantrolene sodium, tizanidine, baclofen) cautiously because these medications are often sedating even in low doses. When specific patterns of spasticity involve particular regions of the body, and when there is associated functional interference (e.g., a "frozen shoulder" that interferes with eating; the wrist and finger flexor contractures that interfere with holding utensils; the ankle extension or equinovarus contracture that interferes with adequate foot and ankle placement during the stance phase of the gait cycle), treatment with injection of botulinum toxin into specific muscle groups by a neurologist or a physiatrist trained to do this procedure should be pursued.

Both rigidity and spasticity can interfere with optimal functioning. They cause shortening of muscles and musculoskeletal soft tissues and predisposition to contracture formation. When severe (e.g., a frozen shoulder), they can disallow functional and controlled movement (e.g., eating, brushing teeth), and encourage poor hygiene in skinfolds (e.g., the armpit) because of lack of access during bathing. Fundamentally, what will reverse and prevent contracture is daily range-of-motion and flexibility programs that can be taught to caregivers by physical and occupational therapists and incorporated into the daily schedule of the individual with dementia.

CREATING A SAFE ENVIRONMENT

As the dementia progresses, the learning ability of the individual will become increasingly finite. The rehabilitation interventions, then, are best directed toward the interpersonal and physical environments. These efforts hopefully improve the sense of control that the caregivers have in an interpersonal situation that can be viewed as relentlessly frustrating and asymmetric.

Creating a safe physical environment can be accomplished inexpensively and with input from home physical therapists, occupational therapists, speech therapists (swallowing), and nurses, and with the purchase of several pieces of durable medical equipment. Any physician can prescribe a home environmental evaluation by the rehabilitation team with the goal of providing the caregiver advice for creating a safe environment. See chapter 14 for a more in-depth discussion of home modifications to increase safety.

MOBILITY (GAIT AND BALANCE) TRAINING AND DURABLE MEDICAL EQUIPMENT (DME)

Mobility training by physical therapy is fundamental to minimize falling risk and prevent falling episodes associated with major injuries such as hip fractures. Dementia is, itself, a risk factor for falling. Fluid, goal-directed movement is dependent on the integrity of an array of cognitive and sensorimotor factors or "intrinsic" factors that interact with the physical environment or "extrinsic" factors to determine safe movement.

As presented in more detail in chapter 11, mobility training focuses on optimizing the intrinsic factors by deconstructing movement into a series of basic and sequential motor tasks that an individual must execute for safe movement: rolling, lying to sitting and vice versa, unsupported sitting balance, sitting to standing and vice versa, transfers or changes in sitting/standing surfaces (e.g., on to and off of toilet, into and out of bed), weight shifting, walking on level surfaces and on nonlevel (e.g., stairs, outdoors) surfaces, integrative balance reactions to environmental challenges (e.g., getting pushed). During mobility training, all sensory systems are being optimized. It is observed that impaired proprioception ("knowing where your body is in space") and impaired vision particularly will compromise movement by disallowing optimal sensory direction of motor control. This, in rehabilitation, is known as sensory-motor integration. Additionally, during mobility training, the focus of strengthening is directed toward improving hip and knee group muscle power as fundamental for maintaining an upright position.

In many situations when mobility is impaired and falling risk is high, an assistive device may be necessary to allow safe walking. From least restrictive to more restrictive, these include straight canes, quad canes, axillary/forearm crutches, hemi-walkers, rolling walkers, and standard walkers. Successful use of the lesser restrictive devices presumes better balance. All of these assistive devices serve two main purposes: provide enhanced sensory feedback to the brain to improve motor control and; decrease energy consumption during walking to conserve strength and endurance. For individuals with FTD, it is essential that they learn the use of an assistive device under the direction of a physical therapist. Most individuals with dementia can procedurally learn to use these devices safely. As the dementia progresses, some individuals with dementia will be unable to initiate and sequence these devices correctly, thus increasing their falling risk.

In addition to assistive devices to support walking, there are other kinds of durable medical equipment (DME) that can optimize mobility when walking is no longer possible:

1. *Wheelchairs*—These should be considered when safe household and/or community ambulation are no longer possible. Their use in individuals with dementia presumes that caregivers are available to propel them and that the individual is not self-propelling. For insurance reimbursement, a physician's

prescription is necessary. This can be taken to a DME vendor who can supply/deliver the wheelchair. The DME vendor will send a certificate of medical necessity (CMN) to the prescribing physician for sign-off after documenting the wheelchair's necessity for household use. For the individual with dementia, foldable, manually controlled lightweight wheelchairs with swing-away or flip-back desk arms, removable/elevating leg rests, and a firm gel/foam combination cushion are recommended. This will allow the caregiver to fold/lift the wheelchair up/down stairs or into/out of the car, the individual to be seated comfortably at a table or desk, the individual's legs to be elevated to facilitate venous return, and a firm base of support to decompress bony weight-bearing sites in the buttocks to allow good sitting posture and prevent pressure sores. Many caregivers find lightweight wheelchairs, weighing between thirty and forty pounds, too heavy to lift. A less supportive, lower cost, and lighter option is a "travel" or "companion" wheelchair weighing twenty to twenty-five pounds.

Motorized scooters or wheelchairs are not recommended for individuals with dementia. Their cognitive deficits will likely interfere with safe driving. Health insurance plans commonly will not pay for "companion control," that is, when a caregiver drives the motorized device.

2. *Hospital beds*—These should be considered when movement in bed and transferring into and out of bed becomes difficult. Health insurance plans commonly reimburse semi-automatic hospital beds, that is, when there is remote control of elevating/lowering the head and foot of the bed and manual control of the height of the bed, with a physician's prescription and sign-off on a CMN via a DME vendor. Fully automatic hospital beds provide remote control of the height of the bed, and can be reimbursed with an additional letter of medical necessity (LMN) from a physician that documents its need for facilitating safe transfers into and out of bed and when a caregiver is unable to control the height of the bed with manual control.

3. *Hoyer lifts*—These should be considered when transfers require at least 50 percent assistance of a caregiver, or less, when the caregiver has health problems. They are manually controlled mobile devices that can be manipulated in the bed-

room and bathroom, and include a sling type of lift. A Hoyer "partner" is an accessory sling made of mesh material that dries quickly if exposed to water in the shower or tub, and can be removed from underneath the dependent individual so that he/she does not have to sit on the sling for a prolonged period of time. These items are insurance reimbursable with a physician's prescription and sign-off on a CMN via a DME vendor.

4. *Commode and raised toilet seats*—These are necessary for a one-floor living arrangement when toileting facilities are not available on the floor where one chooses to live. Even if toileting facilities are available on the same floor, mobility may be impaired, particularly at night time, necessitating their use. The best option is a "three-in-one" commode that can be used at the bedside with its collection component, or the frame and seat can be used as a raised toilet seat without the collection component over the permanent toilet. These items are insurance reimbursable with a physician's prescription and sign-off on a CMN via a DME vendor.

5. *Stair glides / lifts*—These should be considered when ambulation on stairs is no longer safe, and one chooses to continue to live on two floors. Health insurance plans will not reimburse them. They can be rented or purchased from specific vendors who will assess the home environment for their feasibility since they do not fit in all stairways. When installed, an individual will usually require a wheelchair or assistive device for each floor. Purchase or rental of the second set of wheelchairs and assistive devices will require payment out of pocket since health insurance plans will usually not pay for a duplicate set.

Several other caveats about DME are worth mentioning:

1. Many physicians do not know what they are ordering when prescribing DME, and thus depend on the knowledge of a DME vendor. Seek advice from someone on the rehabilitation team who has more experience ordering this equipment—the physiatrist, physical therapist, or occupational therapist.

2. Select a DME vendor who is known to your rehabilitation providers. If the wrong equipment is ordered, or if ongoing

service is needed, a good relationship with a vendor will facilitate equipment return/exchange and/or reimbursement, and repair.

3. The physiatrist has the most experience writing letters of medical necessity with appropriate clinical justification. Information from therapists and DME vendors, based on their own assessments of the individual/environment, can be incorporated into these letters.

ACTIVITIES OF DAILY LIVING (ADL) TRAINING

As summarized in table 2 on page 111, ADL can be categorized as those that one needs to survive inside the household (eating, grooming, bathing, toileting, etc.), and those that are needed to survive in the larger community (shopping, banking, etc.). Supporting optimal control of these skills is usually the focus of occupational therapy and nursing treatments and is discussed in more detail in chapters 12 and 13. Occupational therapists can be particularly useful for teaching individuals with dementia and their caregivers the commonsensical use of adaptive equipment, such as reachers, leg lifters, and built-up utensils, that will serve to conserve energy during the performance of ADL. They can provide practical and resourceful advice on the purchasing of low-cost DME and making changes in the physical environment at home to serve safety and energy conservation. Occupational therapists have specific training in cognitive functions, particularly memory and visuoperception, and can teach the use of procedural strategies to compensate for deficits. They can help caregivers set up structure and consistency in daily life schedules as a fundamental behavioral intervention. They work collaboratively with physical therapists and home nurses on ordering and teaching the proper use of DME and the proper techniques of assisting individuals with basic mobility so that caregivers can prevent injuries to themselves. They are experts in fine motor functioning of the hands to facilitate optimal control when performing/assisting ADL.

ASPIRATION PREVENTION DURING EATING AND SWALLOWING

Aspiration occurs when food, saliva, or gastric contents pass through the larynx and enter the upper airways of the lungs. Aspiration can be life threatening, causing airway obstruction and pneumonia. Swallowing dysfunction, or dysphagia, is the major reason that aspiration occurs. Dysphagia can be observed in dementia for a number of reasons that demonstrate the complexity and elegance of normal swallowing. Swallowing has two major phases, an oral (mouth) phase and a pharyngeal (throat) phase. The oral phase requires voluntary, conscious, and active attention directed toward the pacing of eating, the size of the food/liquid bolus to be ingested, coordination of the mouth and facial muscles and the tongue to chew food and propel food toward the throat. Any problems with focusing and sustaining attention toward these components of the oral phase will increase the risk of aspiration. Furthermore, delayed movement of food/liquid across the mouth toward the throat will increase aspiration risk. The pharyngeal phase is a coordinated, involuntary reflex in which all muscles of the throat except one, the cricopharyngeus, relax to allow passage of food/liquid into the esophagus which anatomically is behind the larynx. The cricopharyngeus controls the epiglottis, and tightens or contracts concurrently while other throat muscles relax, to protect entry of ingested/refluxed/vomited materials into the larynx. An effective cough reflex can propel materials from the upper airways at speeds of up to two hundred miles per hour.

Common symptoms that indicate swallowing difficulties and aspiration include coughing during or after eating/drinking, and a "wet" or gurgling voice during or after eating. Speech therapists have emerged as diagnostic and therapeutic swallowing experts. They can perform a clinical swallowing exam in almost any setting with simple tools. Based on this assessment, they can give practical advice to individuals and their caregivers about operationalizing behavioral strategies during meals to lower aspiration risk and optimize nutritional intake.

When any sort of oral food/liquid ingestion results in aspiration, alternative forms of eating, such as enteral nutritional support (tube feeding) can be considered. The choice for enteral nutrition is complicated, and does not preclude tasting orally ingested foods at least to serve quality-of-life purposes. The work of the speech therapist is discussed in more depth in chapter 10. A discussion about enteral feeding choices is included in chapter 17.

THE DECISION TO STOP DRIVING

The decision to stop driving is a difficult one. Chapter 12 addresses some of the issues about making this decision. It is important to note that physicians are legally obligated to report unsafe drivers to the state registry of motor vehicles. This is best done with open and informed consent of the individual with dementia, and with family support and reassurance, whether the individual agrees or not. When the state registry of motor vehicles is informed that someone is no longer medically able to drive, the burden of responsibility is placed on the individual and the family to prove that he/she is a safe driver by passing certified drivers' training and/or a driving test. Occupational therapists are knowledgeable about such training and testing and can refer to regional subspecialists who manage driving programs. Payment for such driving programs is not reimbursable by health insurance plans.

TABLE I. The Deconditioning Syndrome and Its Preventative Treatments

PRIMARY EFFECTS ON ORGAN SYSTEM	RELATED COMPLICATIONS	PREVENTION AND TREATMENT INTERVENTIONS
Musculoskeletal		
Joint contractures	Impedes self-care and ambulation	Proper positioning of limb, sometimes with static splinting; passive and active range-of-motion exercises with terminal stretch at least twice daily
Muscle weakness and atrophy	Decreased strength, coordination, and balance	Conservative isometric and isotonic strengthening
Osteoporosis	Pathologic fractures	Graduated sitting and standing protocols
Dermatological		
Subcutaneous tissue ischemia	Pressure sores	Optimize nutritional intake
Skin atrophy		Frequent repositioning; specialized mattresses that distribute pressure away from bony prominences; avoiding shear stress when moving patient
Cardiovascular/Pulmonary		
Decreased vascular smooth muscle tone	Postural hypotension	Graduated sitting and standing protocols
Tachyardia at rest and during submaximal exercise with reduced cardiac output	Poor endurance	Graduated ambulation
Hypercoagulable blood	Deep venous thrombosis (DVT); pulmonary embolism	Strengthening excercises (low resistance, high repetition) of the legs

Basilar lung collapse Compromised secretion clearance	Poor ventilation Aspiration	Pneumonia

Genitourinary

Increased calcium clearance Incomplete bladder emptying	Kidney stones Urinary tract infections	Graduated sitting protocols Use of bedside com-mode; regularly scheduled voiding

TABLE 2. Everyday Life Functional Survival Skills

SELF-CARE	MOBILITY	COMMUNICATION
Household		

Eating/drinking
Bathing/grooming
Dressing
Toileting
Bowel/bladder
  control
Sexuality
Cooking
Laundry
Housekeeping
Taking medications
	Bed mobility
	Transfers (bed
	  to chair, chair to
	  toilet, chair to
	  shower seat)
	Ambulation with or
	  without an assistive
	  device, level vs.
	  nonlevel surfaces
	  (stairs)
	Balance
	Wheelchair
	  ambulation and
	  parts management
		Hearing
		Vision
		Orientation
		Attention
		Memory
		Language (talking/
		  gesturing
		Spatial perception
		Organization
		Problem solving

Community		

Shopping
Banking
Managing financial
  and legal affairs
	Nonlevel surface
	  ambulation with or
	  without an assistive
	  device (curbs, ramps,
	  uneven terrain)
	Community
	  wheelchair
	  ambulation
	  (manual vs.
	  motorized)
	Driving
	Using public
	  transportation
	  (bus, taxi,
	  wheelchair, van)
		Using telephones
		Writing, typing, word
		  processing, using
		  computer
		Supervising others in
		  self-care and
		  mobility needs

TABLE 3. The Division of Labor among Rehabilitation Providers

Physiatrist	Medical specialist in rehabilitation; gatekeeper of rehabilitation services; prescribes and monitors therapies and DME; coordinates rehabilitation team.
Physical therapist	Assists in basic mobility skills, including bed mobility, transfers, wheelchair mobility, ambulation; helps with assistive devices for ambulation, including canes, walkers, wheelchairs; manages spasticity with therapeutic exercises; facilitates sensorimotor control, gait training, lower limb bracing (orthotics), balance training.
Occupational therapist	Involved with daily living skills, including feeding, grooming, toileting, dressing, and homemaking; develops fine motor skills of the hand and upper limbs, including splinting (orthotics) and wheelchair accessories; assists with cognitive remediation, especially in the areas of memory and visuoperception.
Speech/swallowing therapist	Provides cognitive remediation as it relates to meaningful communication, especially in the areas of attention, memory, language comprehension, conceptual organization, language production (including nonverbal technologies), and oral-motor articulation; performs swallowing evaluation and treatments, specifically regarding oral-motor and pharyngeal function, aspiration precautions, and oral feeding with different food consistencies.
Nurse	Assists and supervises the patient in using cognitive and functional skills learned in

therapies; educates patient in medication schedule and self-monitoring of medical problems such as diabetes; trains bowel and bladder programs; provides direct wound care and pressure sore prevention.

Nutritionist

Collaborates with physicians and therapists to establish caloric and nutritional requirements; makes recommendations for nutritional support options, depending on the most reliable means of food entry (oral, enteral), and dietary advancement.

Psychologists

Counseling psychologist provides psychotherapeutic treatment of loss reactions, depression, and other mood disorders.

Behavioral psychologist designs and manages behavior strategies and programs (often in concert with medications) aimed at optimizing communication with patients having difficulty with self-monitoring, aggression, poor initiation, and other behaviors that disrupt rehabilitation treatments and social interactions.

Neuropsychologist provides formal assessment of cognitive and intellectual functions; translates cognitive strengths and weaknesses into behaviorally based cognitive remediation strategies.

Orthotist

Fabricates devices that enable motor control and conserve energy consumption during mobility (orthotics), especially of lower limbs.

DME vendor

Supplies and services durable medical equipment based on physician/therapist

	prescription/recommendation with health insurance plan reimbursement or through private payment.
Recreation therapist	Evaluates and remediates motor and cognitive dysfunction in a setting that focuses on leisure activities.
Social worker/case manager	Clarifies social support system, its ability to provide safe and stable emotional support, residential sites, personal care, and transportation; clarifies eligibility and coverage of health and welfare services and health insurance plans; mobilizes resources for coverage of essential health and rehabilitation services with informal and formal care providers acting in complementary roles; provides emotional support for patients and their caregivers; orchestrates appropriate medical, surgical, rehabilitation, and social services, depending on recovery trajectory, treatment priorities, and health insurance/ financial resources.
Caregiver	Supervises and assists in personal care at home; performs preventative/maintenance rehabilitation interventions at home; includes family members, friends, volunteers, neighbors, church community members, and anyone willing to act as an unpaid or informal care provider.

BIBLIOGRAPHY

Robinson, K. M. "Rehabilitation applications in caring for patients with Pick's disease and frontotemporal dementias." *Neurology* 56 (Suppl. 4) (2001): S56–S58.

Robinson, K. M. "Assessing Function." In M. A. Forciea, R. Lavizzo-Mourey, and E. P. Schwab. *Geriatrics Secrets*, 2d ed. Philadelphia: Hanley and Belfus, 2000, pp. 121–28.

Sandel, E. M. et al. "Neurorehabilitation." In *Neurologic and Neurosurgical Emergencies*, edited by J. Cruz. Philadelphia: W. B. Saunders, 1998, pp. 503–46.

Zorowitz, R. D., and K. M. Robinson. "Pathophysiology of dysphagia and aspiration." *Topics in Stroke Rehabilitation* 6, no. 3 (1999): 1–16.

CHAPTER 7

As the Symptoms Progress:
Understanding the Stages of the Disease

CAROL F. LIPPA

While caring for someone who is ill, family members and other caregivers often wish to have information regarding the progression of an individual's disease. After the diagnosis and treatment, inquiries about what to expect in the future are the most frequently asked questions of the physician. Concerns involve three main areas. First, caregivers want information about the rate of disease progression. Then they want to know what symptoms to expect as the disease progresses. Finally, families and other caregivers are interested in ways to slow the rate of disease progression.

RATE OF DISEASE PROGRESSION

Accurate estimates are critical for the patient, family, and physician because treatment decisions are based, in part, upon this information. An individual's rate of progression can be estimated based on his symptoms and signs at specific times after onset, as well as by laboratory and other neurodiagnostic data. However, there is inherent variability in the rate of progression from one patient to another, which we don't understand. In some cases, progression is over months. At the other extreme, cases with duration of more than twenty-five years have been reported. Generally, people live two to ten years from the time of diagnosis. Also, care should be taken to avoid the notion that disease progression for a given individual is solely dependent upon biological aspects of the disease. Controllable psychosocial factors may influence the amount of time that an individual can remain at home and her survival time.

As yet, we can only estimate how rapidly a patient with FTD will progress. One general rule is that many individuals with dementia maintain their disease tempo. Those with a slow onset and few early clinical changes are likely to continue to progress slowly. Those with a more rapid change in behavior or cognition may be more likely to progress quickly. Cognitive rating scales have been used to monitor a patient's rate of disease progression. The most widely used test, the Folstein minimental state examination (MMSE),[1] is a thirty-point test that can provide a rough measure of a dementia patient's rate of progression based on the assumption that most patients will lose two to four points a year unless they are at the extremes of the scale. The MMSE is sometimes used in Alzheimer's disease patients on cholinesterase inhibitors to look for objective evidence of clinical stabilization. An initial decline of more than four points a year is considered rapid; a drop of less than two points a year indicates that an individual is progressing relatively slowly. However, caution must be used if the physician administers the MMSE to the FTD patient, because it may not assess all their symptoms. The personality changes and changes in energy and behavior that are common in FTD are not evaluated, so a patient with obvious behavioral worsening may appear to be stable on the MMSE. Also, some FTD patients have prominent problems with language. The MMSE is heavily language based, so the frontotemporal individuals with language problems may acquire scores that overestimate their rate of progression.

When trying to determine whether an individual will progress quickly, the presence or absence of other neurological symptoms is helpful. Patients with problems involving chewing, swallowing, or voice volume tend to do poorly. However, before deciding that the prognosis is poor, you will want to assess the reasons for these symptoms. If the patient doesn't eat because he is inattentive or because she lacks the initiative to feed herself, prognosis is more favorable if strategies can be developed to circumvent the problem. Alternately, loss of ability to control the mouth, throat, and tongue suggests that the disease has involved deep brain regions that are spared until the late disease stages.

Dementia patients with movement problems may progress at a more rapid rate than those who show no problems with movement. Patients who have stiffness, slowness, and tremors tend to have rapid rates of progression. This is also, in part, because the control centers for movement are in deep brain regions that are not usually affected early in the disease. Another reason is that sometimes frontotemporal dementia occurs in association with amyotrophic lateral sclerosis (ALS). ALS patients have difficulty with strength in addition to frontotemporal symptoms. The course is rapid because the motor symptoms worsen quickly; most die from breathing problems within several years.

If there are early problems with movement, it is important to first rule out an associated condition that has features of frontotemporal dementia. These disorders include progressive supranuclear palsy and corticobasal degeneration. A neurologist can help you with these diagnoses, particularly early or in the midportion of the disease course. It is important to make this distinction because the symptoms these patients develop may differ from pure FTD. Also, there may be medications available to help treat the motor symptoms of progressive supranuclear palsy and corticobasal degeneration. Once a patient has advanced disease and becomes mute or immobile, it is more difficult for the physician to determine the diagnosis since many dementia subtypes look similar in the end stages.

One final complicating factor in assessing the rate of disease progression is that the disease onset in FTD can be difficult to assess. Symptoms are caused by a progressive loss of brain cells and brain cell processes in the frontal and temporal lobes. Biologically, the disease process starts years before the individual shows any symptoms of the disease. Symptoms are often insidious at onset. Furthermore, many of the symptoms that patients with FTD experience are initially exaggerations of previous behaviors. Sometimes they are confused with signs of a midlife crisis. These factors make it difficult to date the exact time of disease onset and thus make the rate of progression more difficult to determine.

WHAT TO EXPECT OVER TIME

The second question about progression is what symptoms to expect as the disease progresses. Patients with frontotemporal dementia are more complicated than those with other diseases due to the wide variety of symptoms they experience and their tendency to go through different phases during the disease process. When compared with Alzheimer's disease patients, those with FTD have different initial symptoms. They may also develop symptoms at an earlier age than comparable patients with other types of dementia. Binetti et al. determined that FTD subjects are more likely to experience language problems or personality change as initial symptoms. Alzheimer's disease patients usually present to the physician with memory problems. Patients with FTD often do worse on cognitive tests (except for visuospatial tests) and scales of activities of daily functioning than Alzheimer's disease patients at the time they are initially assessed by a physician.[2] They show a more rapid progression of language problems and a more rapid decline on global measures of dementia than Alzheimer's disease patients.[3]

There are certain symptoms that can be anticipated as frontotemporal dementia progresses. One is difficulty with language. When the left side of the brain is involved, the affected individual has trouble with language-based tasks such as speech fluency, word finding, sentence length, writing, and understanding language. Most FTD patients develop language problems, especially speech expression problems, at some point during their clinical course. If language difficulties are not a presenting symptom, they should be expected to develop as the disease progresses. Many individuals with FTD become mute as the disease advances.

Energy and initiative are common problems in FTD and may also be anticipated at some point in the disease. Restlessness is not uncommon, especially in the earlier disease stages. Changes in energy often occur; apathy and inertia can be major problems in FTD patients as the disease progresses.

INFLUENCING DISEASE PROGRESSION

Cholinesterase inhibitors, including donepezil, rivastigmine, and galantamine, are sometimes used to help stabilize the cognitive symptoms in frontotemporal dementia subjects. These agents may give the individual a degree of symptomatic benefit, but they have not been shown to have an independent effect to slow down the rate of disease progression. Their use should be discussed with the individual's physician; there are differing opinions about the effectiveness and safety of these agents. If prescribed, these medications should be monitored carefully since frontotemporal dementia patients may be more likely to experience side effects from them. (See chapter 5 for more information.)

Medications can sometimes target specific symptoms, especially the behavioral problems. They may enable affected individuals to remain in a less restrictive environment for extended periods of time. Behavioral interventions are probably more effective than medications for many of the symptoms these individuals experience. No medication provides a major benefit on language problems in these individuals.

Nonprescription medications have been shown to impact disease course in related conditions. Studies demonstrate that high doses of vitamin E (2,000 international units a day) helps improve outcome in Alzheimer's disease.[4] There have been no studies focusing on its effectiveness in FTD. Since high doses of vitamin E may increase bruising or bleeding tendencies, the dose administered should be discussed with the individual's physician.

Although there are no studies proving the effect of physical and mental activity on the symptoms of frontotemporal dementia, there are studies of Alzheimer's dementia subjects indicating that those who remain physically and mentally active fare better over time. As such, it's reasonable to encourage activity. The specific physical/ mental activities do not matter. However, to avoid frustrating the individual, care should be taken to avoid mental or physical challenges that she can no longer do easily. It is best to select and encourage increased involvement in activities that the individual enjoys and can still participate in effectively.

Frontotemporal dementia doesn't often cause death directly, because the brain areas most severely affected are those involved with thinking rather than those that regulate the heart and breathing muscles. As the disease advances, individuals become less mobile. Once they stop walking they are susceptible to developing infections, particularly pneumonia and urinary tract infections. As they lose fitness their body is less able to clear infections. This is the most common cause of death. Elderly individuals with FTD may also die from cancer, myocardial infarctions (heart attacks), and other diseases that affect the elderly.

Overall, there is marked variability in symptom progression in frontotemporal dementia. If the duration of symptoms can be estimated, the rate of progression often remains the same. Those with difficulty moving or swallowing may have a more rapid clinical course. Affected individuals are often younger at onset than Alzheimer's disease patients, and their symptoms are different, especially in the early stages of the disease. Most frontotemporal dementia patients develop problems with language and energy at some point in the disease, and problems with thinking (attention, concentration, problem solving, and behavior) can be severe. Medications and behavioral strategies may be used to influence an individual's ability to remain in an optimal environment.

NOTES

1. M. F. Folstein, S. E. Folstein, and P. R. McHugh, "Mini-mental state—A practical method for grading the cognitive state of patients for the clinician," *Journal of Psychiatric Research* 12 (1975): 189–98.

2. G. Binetti et al., "Differences between Pick disease and Alzheimer disease in clinical appearance and rate of cognitive decline," *Archives of Neurology* 57 (2000): 225–32.

3. Ibid.

4. M. Sano et al., "A controlled trial of selegiline, alpha-tocopherol, or both as treatment for Alzheimer's disease," *New England Journal of Medicine* 336 (2000): 1216–22.

CHAPTER 8

An Immortal Legacy:
The Human Impact of Biomedical Research and Autopsy

JENNIFER M. FARMER, VIRGINIA M.-Y. LEE, AND JOHN Q. TROJANOWSKI

THE IMPORTANCE OF AN AUTOPSY

A rigorously conducted autopsy or postmortem investigation to establish a proximal (actual) cause of death and to identify other disorders that contributed to the failure and compromised health status of an individual afflicted by disease has been called the "ultimate medical consultation." Also, it serves important roles in the oversight or monitoring of the quality and adequacy of the medical care a patient has received during life by confirming, clarifying, and correcting clinical diagnoses. Therefore, autopsies often provide unique and critical information on the relative effectiveness of novel versus established medications, operative procedures, and other disease interventions.

Autopsy studies further serve to document disease rates and provide data for local and national population registries concerning changing trends in mortality, infection, and other health care concerns. Epidemiological autopsy data also are essential for accurate estimates of the true occurrence rates of existing and well known— as well as underdiagnosed and newly emerging—diseases. Autopsy data can also provide important information leading to the identification of new or unsuspected diseases. Examples of disorders that are better understood now compared to a few decades ago, as a result of autopsy studies, include Legionnaires' and Alzheimer's disease, sudden infant death, toxic shock, and acquired immunodeficiency syndromes. Indeed, a growing body of data from an increasing number of postmortem studies of FTDs, the focus of this chapter, is providing a much clearer picture of these relentlessly progressive and ultimately fatal neurodegenerative disorders. This surge in data on FTDs suggests that they may be more common than previously reported.

Other socially beneficial purposes served by autopsies include (1) biomedical research to discover the causes and better treatments for disease, (2) detecting the health-related consequences of a wide variety of occupational exposures, and (3) delivery of life-saving treatments for living individuals by playing a key role in the acquisition, preservation, and donation of human skin, bone, cornea, and other organs for transplantation therapy. In medicolegal cases, autopsy establishes the means and manner of death. For instance, autopsies have helped link fatal poisoning to product tampering in several over-the-counter drug preparations. Autopsy once played a major role in medical school education, but because of declining autopsy rates in hospitals, use of this important teaching medium for medical students is dwindling throughout the United States.

A BRIEF HISTORY OF AUTOPSY

The Greek word "autopsia" means "to see with one's own eyes." Ancient Greeks focused their attention on an imbalance of fluids and vapors or humors, rather than organs and anatomic structures, as causes of disease. Egyptian embalmers of the Early, Middle, and Late Kingdoms had knowledge of human anatomy. They routinely removed organs in their work to mummify or preserve the bodies of deceased pharaohs and other members of the ruling elite for the afterlife. But, these highly skilled anatomists did not convey many of their observations in writing to the scientific community. Prompted by new autopsy-derived data, Erasistratus abandoned the popular humoral theory of disease developed earlier by Hippocrates, and Erasistratus is generally credited for making the association of organ change and disease by carrying out dissections of the human body as long ago as 300 B.C.E.

In the European Middle Ages, the church did not generally

accept postmortem dissections, although popes did direct autopsies to be performed to search for a cause of the plague, which decimated large populations at that time. It was not until the Renaissance in the fifteenth century that the autopsy became an established investigative method and began to play a significant role in advancing medical science. Subsequently, by the eighteenth century, scientists and clinicians were carrying out comprehensive studies to correlate clinical and autopsy data at leading medical centers throughout Europe.

By the mid-nineteenth century the social and medical benefits of the autopsy were widely appreciated. Following informed consent of authorized family members, individuals dying in academic health centers as recently as the mid-twentieth century in the United States had approximately a 50 percent chance of being autopsied to determine the cause of death. In fact, the percentage was higher in many European countries, where permission to conduct an autopsy on a decedent was the socially and legally accepted assumption unless the family specifically declined to allow it.

Today in the United States, the autopsy rate in most academic health centers hovers around 10 percent, and is still falling. Autopsies are rarely performed in for-profit hospitals, and this has occurred for several reasons. First, in 1971, after the Joint Commission for the Accreditation of Health Organizations dropped the recommended 20 percent autopsy rate for hospitals, there was a diminished emphasis on autopsy as part of the medical school curriculum at many universities. Second, the growing success and emphasis on technical advances (e.g., medical imaging) and many advances in experimental research led to a decreasing reliance on postmortem examination as a means of gaining new knowledge. This was despite the fact that the clinical or antemortem diagnostic error rates determined through autopsy examinations has remained constant at around 12 percent for the past several decades.

Since autopsies are not revenue-producing activities, but cost approximately $3,000 per case, they have been subject to cutbacks in an era of healthcare cost containment. If the death of a patient occurs outside a facility where they had been monitored by clinicians, there are charges for the transportation of the body to the clinicians' facility for postmortem examination. This charge (which can range from a few to several hundred dollars) may be an overwhelming financial burden for families that influences their decision to decline an autopsy on their loved one. In addition, physician attitudes have changed such that they may be less inclined to request an autopsy out of a fear of increased risk of medical liability. Despite the lack of concrete evidence for this, these factors have led to inadequate numbers of pathologists (physicians specializing in laboratory medicine) to perform autopsies. Finally, recent trends in scientific research have focused less on innovative findings from postmortem studies. This also has contributed to a declining interest of the biomedical research community in autopsy studies and data derived from them.

Religious beliefs and philosophical views of different ethnic groups have profoundly influenced the extent to which diverse cultures in the United States as well as in regions throughout the world value the social and medical benefits of autopsy studies. However, many religions (e.g., Christianity, Hinduism, Buddhism, Taoism, Confucianism, Shintoism) have no specific religious tenets that prohibit the postmortem examination of deceased members of their faith. Jewish religious authorities have permitted autopsies since the eighteenth century, although Orthodox Judaism forbids its followers from consenting to an autopsy. This also is the view of Muslims.

THE AUTOPSY PROCESS

Currently, in the United States, a family member of the deceased must give written or verbal permission for an autopsy of their loved one, except in certain medicolegal cases that fall under the jurisdiction of the municipal medical examiner's office. The spouse of the deceased individual usually has the overriding right to give consent for an autopsy, but state laws vary regarding which family member can exercise this right if there is no surviving spouse. Consent for complete postmortem examination is obtained in approximately 75 percent of autopsies. Family members may limit their consent for autopsy to specified organs or body parts (such as the trunk or brain only). These "problem-targeted" (diagnosis-oriented) autopsies can answer specific questions regarding one or more of the patient's clinical diagnoses. In contrast to a complete autopsy, in which all major organs are removed and examined, a limited autopsy may include inspection of the organs without removal of any of them. It also may permit the microscopic examination of small biopsy samples from selected organs.

While the foregoing applies to most autopsies, the ground rules are different for forensic autopsies that are conducted for medico-legal reasons. Briefly, forensic medicine refers to the scientific application of medical knowledge to resolve legal problems. Medicolegal deaths refer to deaths that must be investigated in accordance with state and federal laws, such as unexpected or violent deaths, suspicious deaths, etc. In a forensic autopsy, which refers to postmortem studies focused on determining the cause of death for legal reasons, several distinctions need to be made to fully explain the death. For example, the cause of death in a forensic autopsy report refers to the disease or injury that is responsible for the death. The proximate cause of death is the event or disease that started the sequence of events ending in the death of the individual, and the immediate cause of death includes complications and terminal events that result from the proximate cause of death.

Although similar issues are addressed in academic or nonforensic autopsies, *the emphasis in autopsies conducted for research studies is on determining not only the key diagnoses, but also the disease mechanisms that led to the death of the patient—including the underlying physiological or pathological process.* However, since there are many poorly understood diseases that remain to be investigated, as exemplified by FTDs, it may not be possible to specify this in all cases. Thus, in the case of an individual afflicted with a neurodegenerative disease such as FTD that is associated with progressive cognitive impairments, the patient may be determined to have FTD as a proximate cause of death, pneumonia as the immediate cause, and infection as the mechanism of the individual's death.

A complete postmortem examination begins with careful evaluation of the exterior of the body and includes notations of wounds, scars, and any other skin abnormalities. Dissection begins with a small abdominal incision to enable inspection of the chest and abdominal organs, which the pathologist removes and further dissects to examine organ parenchyma, ducts, blood vessels, and lumens. In most autopsies, the pathologist dissects all organs and samples small portions of each organ for microscopic analysis of evident abnormalities. The pathologist examines the brain in a similar manner, following removal through an incision made at the back of the head, but the face and limbs are never dissected in an academic or nonforensic autopsy. Hence, even a sophisticated pathologist cannot surmise whether an autopsy has or has not been performed on someone viewed at a traditional open-casket funeral service.

After overall examination, the pathologist studies each organ and records its weight and measurements as well as other salient normal or abnormal features. Following fixation to preserve the tissue samples for subsequent investigations, the pathologist uses a microscope to study samples selected for histological analysis. Additionally, as the case dictates, the most critical diagnostic information may come from biochemical or microbiological analysis of small tissue samples or fluids. In selected cases, toxicology studies may be performed to rule out drug- or toxin-induced medical disorders. Finally, all of the pertinent data from the autopsy studies are summarized into a coherent technical report of the patient's illness. This is correlated with the autopsy findings to reconcile both data sets into a lucid account of how all of the pathological findings contributed to the clinical manifestations of the patient and led to his/her demise. An autopsy and the formal report have several benefits to the family including:

- clarification of the relevant diagnoses
- reassurance from knowing the cause of death and relief of any guilt when a patient dies unexpectedly or from poorly understood diseases
- knowledge that the appropriate care has been provided for the patient during his/her illness
- identification of genetic conditions that might have contributed to disease onset or progression
- knowledge about any contagious diseases the patient might have had so that appropriate measures can be taken to protect the family members
- advancement of medical research to develop better or new therapies for diseases

Common concerns about giving consent for an autopsy are:

- body disfigurement, mutilation, and delaying of funeral
- lack of information about the reasons for autopsy and the benefits it provides to families and society

- objection from other family members, based on religious background, family dynamics, or lack of understanding
- cost and logistics

These issues should be discussed with your healthcare providers and researchers, family members, and support resources (e.g., clergy) to help make a decision that is good for you and your family. One common misconception is that the clinical diagnoses of a deceased loved one are correct, therefore an autopsy is not necessary. But, it is known through autopsies conducted at academic health centers over many decades that clinical diagnoses are incorrect approximately 12 percent of the time, and for FTDs and other neurodegenerative dementias, the *only* accurate way to make a correct diagnosis is through an autopsy. Oftentimes, another concern is that family members may feel the deceased or family has suffered enough and that an autopsy will only serve to prolong the suffering. However, information gleaned from an autopsy often promotes closure among family members. Furthermore, families should be reassured that a pathologist is a highly skilled member of the healthcare team who will perform the autopsy with respect and concern for the dignity of the deceased. Organs will be removed for study through the incisions mentioned above and will be hidden by clothing, thus allowing for an open-casket funeral service. Additionally, concerns about interference with funeral arrangements are unwarranted, since the removal and inspection of organs at autopsy takes only one to two hours and arrangements can be made to facilitate timely examination.

The complete analysis of samples removed at autopsy may require the expertise of several pathologists with special knowledge of diseases involving the heart, brain, kidneys, and other relevant organ systems. It may take several weeks for all of the relevant studies to be completed and for the final autopsy report to be compiled, but the family can request a copy of this technical document. Although an autopsy report may be challenging for the nonspecialist to understand, the family can seek consultation with the patient's doctor and/or the pathologists involved in the postmortem studies.

RESEARCH ON HUMAN TISSUES AND BODILY FLUIDS

While the previous considerations about autopsy do not apply in exactly the same manner to biological samples (e.g., blood, tissue biopsies, bodily fluids) from living patients, many considerations do. Some of these considerations are:

- the need for informed consent from the individual or family member for obtaining and conducting studies on the samples
- the critical importance of such samples for determining an accurate diagnosis of the patient's condition
- to further biomedical research and learn more about the underlying causes of disease and developing therapies

The myths or misunderstandings about what is involved when patients and family members provide biological samples to medical researchers need to be addressed. With increased understanding of the issues, patients and families have provided biological samples from living and deceased individuals, contributing substantially to basic and clinical studies of FTD and related disorders. This is driving biomedical progress in neurodegenerative dementias with breathtaking speed.

IMPACT OF BIOMEDICAL AND AUTOPSY RESEARCH ON FTD

Translating biological research studies into clinical care that impacts the quality of medical care and treatment received by an individual is the ultimate goal and challenge. Knowledge that has been gained through autopsy-based research has advanced biomedical research in neuropathology (the study of brain, spinal cord, and nerve cells) and our understanding of FTDs. This has most dramatically been proven in the ability to identify unique clinical and diagnostic features, syndromes, and subtypes among FTDs, as reviewed in chapter 2.

Brain tissue studies of neurodegenerative conditions have led to the realization that most of these conditions have unique or hallmark brain findings, such as abnormal accumulations of specific proteins in defined regions and/or loss or shrinkage of brain tissue in defined regions of the brain. Table 1 on page 134 provides a listing of neurodegenerative conditions and the specific protein found to be abnormal in the brain. For example, in Parkinson's disease it was shown that the protein alpha-synuclein is the building block of the Lewy bodies in neurons (nerve cells or brain cells).

Common neurodegenerative diseases like AD, which has been the focus of intense research for many years, have paved the way for the more recent work on the FTDs. Enormous progress has been made to improve the reliability and accuracy of methods and procedures for the antemortem and postmortem diagnosis of AD and other dementias. This has led to the recognition that AD is a disorder caused by multiple genetic and environmental influences and with a set of distinct clinical and postmortem features that distinguish AD from other dementias.

In AD, characteristic abnormalities seen in the brain are senile plaques and neurofibrillary tangles, along with shrinkage or cell death in specific regions of the brain, beginning in the hippocampus and amygdala, then spreading to the cortex (outer regions). Senile plaques are a buildup of amyloid, a protein which prevents brain cells from communicating with a neighboring cell. Through the combined efforts of neuropathology and genetic research, a gene that is responsible for forming the senile plaques was identified: *amyloid precursor protein (APP)* gene. A fundamental contribution that came from studies of biological samples containing DNA from living and deceased patients and family members was the identification of disease-associated mutations in genes on chromosomes 21 (the *APP* gene), 14, and 1 (the presenilin 1 and 2 genes, respectively) that cause familial or inherited AD. Based on these new findings, researchers have been able to establish animal models of AD.

As a result of improvements in the standardization of the clinical and neuropathological diagnosis of AD, it has been possible to conduct more rigorous research on well-characterized AD patients, including studies of tissues and other biological samples or fluids from these individuals. Significantly, this has enabled scientists to have access to well-characterized patient samples, including blood, cerebral spinal fluid (the fluid produced in the brain that surrounds it), and postmortem brain tissues, for basic and clinical research to identify more accurate biomarkers of AD. Moreover, other neurodegenerative dementias previously confused with AD, including FTDs, now can be distinguished more reliably from AD. Research discoveries in AD and other neurodegenerative conditions are likely to have a significant impact on our understanding of FTDs and advancements toward therapies.

Insights into the composition of the neurofibrillary tangles of AD have directly advanced our knowledge of FTDs. These tangles contain abnormal forms of tau protein. Normal tau has an important function in the brain cell: it is the crosspiece between microtubules. One can think of microtubules as train tracks and tau as the railroad ties used to hold the track together properly. The microtubules and tau are important for sending information through the cell. Nerve cells can be very long; therefore, a secure transmitting structure is important. When tau is abnormal it causes the microtubules to twist and take on a helical shape, thus the term "helical filaments" is used, as it describes the appearance of the abnormal tau proteins under the microscope. Abnormal tau is like having a broken rail tie that causes the track to be unsecure. Just as a train cannot travel down an unsecure track, information in the cell cannot travel down a microtubule that is twisted or comes apart. When information cannot travel through the cell, it is more likely to die than the surrounding unaffected cells. Abnormal tau in the brain has been documented in many neurodegenerative conditions, including FTD. As a group, these conditions are commonly referred to as "tauopathies." Table 2 on page 135 contains a list of some of the conditions characterized by abnormal tau in the brain. Mutations in the gene that encodes tau (*MAPT* gene) have been shown to cause familial forms of FTD. This is discussed in chapter 3 in more detail.

More recently, a sense of optimism about breakthroughs in understanding FTDs is growing as more investigators seek to conduct research on this complex group of disorders. It is now appreciated that many FTDs are characterized by brain degeneration, primarily in the frontal and temporal lobes, linked to accumulations of tau-containing neurofibrillary tangles. As in AD, these tangles are caused by abnormal tau protein that aggregates in the neurons. Research has further defined the abnormal forms of tau (based on length and additional chemical tags, or phosphorylation). The presence of specific forms of tau in different variants of FTDs has recently been documented and used for diagnostic purposes. Some individuals thought to have FTD, based on clinical features and frontal and temporal brain loss, did not have abnormal accumulations of tau or other readily identifiable proteins. The neuropathologic term used to describe this group is "Dementia Lacking Distinct Histopathological features." Indeed, this growing interest in FTDs prompted an international group of experts on clinical and neuropathological aspects of FTDs to re-examine criteria for the diagnosis of FTD at a meeting entitled "The Frontotemporal Dementia and Pick's Disease Criteria Conference" held at the National Institutes of Health in Bethesda, Maryland, on July 7, 2000. Building upon the substantial scientific literature on these disorders, the goals of the conference were to update previous FTD diagnostic criteria, taking into account recent research advances, to refine guidelines for the clinical and neuropathological diagnosis of FTD. Table 3 on pages 135–36 contains a brief synopsis of the neuropathologic diagnostic criteria used to distinguish different types of FTD.

Of significance to caregivers and the families of FTD patients is the fact that most criteria for the diagnosis of neurodegenerative diseases require correlation of clinical data obtained from patients followed during life in addition to the neuropathological findings gleaned from postmortem studies of the brain and other organs. Indeed, academic centers that pursue studies of FTDs and other neurodegenerative disorders are obligated to adhere to strict protocols to retain their funding from granting agencies. Thus, for these reasons, it is recommended that families seek out institutions that have followed the protocols when they are contemplating plans for brain donation. While there is much more that needs to be learned about the mechanisms of brain degeneration in the diverse forms of FTDs before research findings can be translated into focused drug discovery efforts, meetings of experts on neurodegenerative diseases—such as the one mentioned above that involves a multidisciplinary group of clinical and basic scientists—will help foster more rapid advances into the causes and treatments of FTDs. However, this will require the continued access of investigators to relevant human biological samples from living and deceased FTD patients for research.

CONCLUSION

In summary, donation of biological samples through autopsy of deceased patients, or by other means from living subjects, satisfies altruistic needs and the personal interests of individuals. These magnanimous acts of patients and their families leave an immortal legacy to future generations of human beings, since knowledge obtained from research on these samples will have lasting benefits far into the future.

TABLE I. Neurodegenerative Diseases Characterized by Lesions in the Brain That Are Formed by Proteins

Disease	Lesions	Protein
Alzheimer's disease	Senile plaques	Amyloid
	Neurofibrillary tangles	Tau
	Lewy bodies	a-Synuclein
Amyotrophic lateral sclerosis	Spheroids	Neurofilaments
Dementia with Lewy bodies	Lewy bodies	a-Synuclein
Multiple system atrophy	Glial cytoplasmic inclusions	a-Synuclein
Parkinson's disease	Lewy bodies	a-Synuclein
Prion diseases (Creutzfeldt-Jakob disease)	Senile plaques	Prions
Tauopathies (FTDs)	Neurofibrillary tangles	Tau

TABLE 2. Neurodegenerative Conditions
That Have Tau Pathology

- Alzheimer's disease
- Down's syndrome
- Prion diseases (Creutzfeldt-Jakob disease)
- Amyotrophic lateral sclerosis/Parkinsonism-dementia complex
- Argyophilic grain dementia

- **Corticobasal degeneration**
- **Frontotemporal dementia/Parkinsonism linked to chromosone 17**

- Hallervorden-Spatz disease
- Multiple system atrophy
- Nieman-Pick disease type C

- **Pick's disease**

- **Progressive supranuclear palsy**

   Note: This is not a complete listing, and the diseases in bold have tau pathology as the predominant or exclusive brain lesions.

TABLE 3. Current Classification of Frontotemporal Dementias Based on Neuropathological Data

1. When the predominant brain abnormalities are tau inclusions in brain cells with a loss of nerve cells and accumulations predominantly of the smaller forms of brain tau, the most likely diagnoses are:
   - Pick's disease
   - FTD with Parkinsonism linked to chromosome 17 (FTDP-17)
   - Other

2. When the predominant brain abnormalities are tau inclusions in brain cells with a loss of nerve cells and accumulations predominantly of the larger forms of brain tau, the most likely diagnoses are:

- Corticobasal degeneration
- Progressive supranuclear palsy
- FTDP-17
- Other

3. When the predominant brain abnormalities are tau inclusions in brain cells with a loss of nerve cells and accumulations of both the larger and smaller forms of brain tau, the most likely diagnoses are:
   - Neurofibrillary tangle dementia
   - FTDP-17
   - Other

4. When the predominant brain abnormalities are nerve cell loss without tau or other inclusions in brain cells and there is little or no detectable tau proteins in the brain, the most likely diagnoses are:
   - FTD lacking distinctive histopathology
   - Other

5) When the predominant brain abnormalities are nerve cell loss in frontal and temporal lobes of the brain with inclusions in brain cells that contain a protein known as ubiquitin, but not tau, neurofilament, or alpha-synuclein the most likely diagnoses are:
   - FTD with motor neuron disease type inclusions
   - Other

Table Legend

These criteria may be used by pathologists to further define the specific type of FTD. However, only probabilistic statements can be made about the causal relationships between neuropathological findings and clinical manifestations of a patient's disease. It is not entirely clear how neurodegenerative diseases cause the dysfunction and death of brain cells or specific neuropsychiatric symptoms. Further, the correlation of neuropathological findings with FTD in a patient does not prove a cause-and-effect relationship, since more than one brain abnormality may contribute to the manifestations of dementia. Finally, the neuropathological findings alone cannot establish that the patient had FTD in the absence of documented clinical information (presented in chapter 2).

NOTE

Virginia M.-Y. Lee is the John H. Ware 3rd Chair of Alzheimer's disease research at the University of Pennsylvania. Work done in the laboratories of the authors is supported by grants from the National Institute of Aging of the National Institutes of Health and the Alzheimer's Association. We also thank our many collaborators and past as well as current members of the Center for Neurodegenerative Disease Research (CNDR) for contributions to the research from CNDR summarized here. Finally, the support of the families of our patients has made this research possible.

The University of Pennsylvania Alzheimer's Disease Center (ADC) was funded by the NIA in 1991 and it is the first and only NIA-funded ADC in the Delaware Valley (for more information on AD and details on the Penn ADCC, see http://www.med.upenn.edu/CNDR/ and http://www.med.upenn.edu/ADC/).

BIBLIOGRAPHY

Clark, C. M., and J. Q. Trojanowski, eds. *Neurodegenerative Dementias: Clinical Features and Pathological Mechanisms.* New York: McGraw-Hill, 2000.

Hyman, B. T., and J. Q. Trojanowski. "Editorial on consensus recommendations for the postmortem diagnosis of Alzheimer's disease from the National Institute on Aging and the Reagan Institute Working Group on Diagnostic Criteria for the Neuropathological Assessment of Alzheimer's Disease." *Journal of Neruopathology and Experimental Neurology* 56 (1997): 1095–97.

McKhann, G. M. et al., "Clinical and pathological diagnosis of frontotemporal dementia: Report of Work Group on Frontotemporal Dementia and Pick's Disease." *Archives of Neurology* 58 (2001): 1803–1809.

"National Institute on Aging and Reagan Institute Working Group on Diagnostic Criteria for the Neuropathological Assessment of Alzheimer's Disease. Consensus recommendations for the postmortem diagnosis of Alzheimer's disease." *Neurobiology of Aging* 18, no. 4S (1997): S1–S2.

Souder, E., and J. Q. Trojanowski. "Autopsy: Cutting away the myths." *Journal of Neuroscience Nursing* 24 (1992): 134–39.

Trojanowski, J. Q. "Alzheimer's disease centers and the Dementias of Aging program of the National Institute on Aging: A brief overview." *Journal of Alzheimer's Disease* 3 (2001): 249–51.

——. "Tauists, Baptists, Syners, apostates, and new data." *Annals of Neurology.* (2002): 263–65.

——. "Emerging Alzhiemer's disease therapies: Focusing on the future." *Neurobiology of Aging* 23 (2002): 985–90.

Trojanowski, J. Q., and D. W. Dickson. "Update on the neuropathological diagnosis of frontotemporal dementias." *Journal of Neuropathology and Experimental Neurology* 60 (2001): 1123–26.

CHAPTER 9

Searching for the Answers:

The Future of Research and Clinical Care

JORDAN GRAFMAN

By the time you read this chapter, I hope you are encouraged that so many healthcare professionals and researchers are devoted to the care and study of patients with FTD. Advances in our understanding of the genetics, neurochemistry, neuropathology, neuropsychology, and epidemiology of FTD are occurring almost monthly, enabling doctors to identify and diagnose FTD earlier, classify potential subtypes of FTD better, and to verify with greater certainty the diagnosis at autopsy.

Much slower progress is being made in developing potential treatments for FTD. FTD is a label that comes with a set of restraints. Drug companies refrain from developing new drugs for FTD since they will gain fewer, if any, profits from the development of a drug for a comparatively rare dementia. Researchers refrain from studying FTD since grant monies are generally more available for the study of more common neurological disorders (such as Alzheimer's disease). Clinicians only occasionally see patients with FTD and therefore have less experience in their clinical care and management.

All of these scenarios make it less likely that a medical intervention such as a new drug or treatment will be developed in a short period of time. That is why, in the case of FTD, it is very important for advocates to organize, press their agenda, and be outspoken in their efforts to obtain public and private funding for research into

FTD. But if there were increased funding available, where would we want to allocate it so that it facilitates the scientific race for a cure for FTD?

There is no doubt that a better understanding of the molecular genetic pathways that fail in FTD would lead to new ideas about how to identify, treat, and prevent it. Molecular genetic technique-driven research is a hopeful and common contemporary strategy used for a host of diseases and what spurred federal and private funding for sequencing the human genome. Molecular genetic studies require that FTD be studied in families in which the disease runs or with the use of hypothesis-driven strategies in sporadic cases of FTD. In some diseases, patients may have a genetic susceptibility for developing a neurological disorder but need an environmental exposure (e.g., exposure to a toxin, smoking, stress) to trigger the onset of the disorder. Neuroepidemiological studies of FTD are badly needed so that any environmental triggers that exist can be identified. Such studies may pinpoint, for example, which specific environmental exposures are associated with the development of FTD. These studies require multicenter involvement because of the relatively small number of FTD patients that travel for their evaluation to research centers, a theme that will be returned to later. There is a cascade of biological events traveling from the chromosome to protein development and regulation to cell function and eventually ensuring a healthy neural environment in the brain. While scientists are beginning to understand where the failure is in this pathway (e.g., abnormal tau protein aggregation), the trigger for the failure remains unknown at this time.

Since FTD causes degeneration of neurons in specific areas of the brain, one result is that certain neurochemicals are disproportionately diminished in FTD. Scientists have found that serotonin and dopamine transmission is abnormal in FTD. Few studies, however, have been conducted to determine the sensitivity or specificity of the change in neurotransmitter function in FTD. Why might it be important to increase the number of studies in this area? Until a treatment for FTD is developed, the next best strategy might be to replace either the chemicals (or neurons—see below) in the affected areas, a strategy that has had some success in the stability of some symptoms of Alzheimer's disease. This would effectively amount to symptomatic treatment. But, keeping a patient stable over a relatively short period of time (months) amounts to improved quality of life for the family and financial savings to the healthcare system. Another way to approach this issue is to simply begin administering medications that have been used to ameliorate symptoms when treating similar neurotransmitter abnormalities in other disorders, ranging from depression to attention deficit disorder. Given the relatively few numbers of patients seen at any one research center, it would be advantageous to conduct multicenter drug studies using the model developed by the Parkinson's Study Group.

What about figuring out a strategy to promote new neural development in order to replace the dying neurons in the frontal and temporal lobes in FTD? Easier said than done. It is one thing to target a small cluster of dying neurons in a small part of the brain and then with specialized surgery to introduce neural stem cells to replace the dying cells. It is a much greater challenge to distribute millions of neural stem cells to the wide swath of cerebral cortex that is damaged in FTD. Even if it could be done today, the neurons would have to be trained via stimulation by the environment to organize themselves in a way that resembled the usual organization of the neurons in that cortex so they could function normally. It is unclear this could be accomplished in the case of the complex cognitive processes mediated by the frontal and temporal lobes, as opposed to retraining simple motor skills. This is, however, a promising area of research, but to bridge the gulf between promising basic research in animals and successful human applications will probably require, at a minimum, many decades.

Structural and functional neuroimaging are important techniques used in the diagnostic process. The ability to obtain clear and precise images of regional atrophic brain structure allows earlier and more definitive diagnoses of FTD to be made. The earlier the diagnosis, the more likely success a drug treatment, for example, may have. Structural imaging allows us to measure the size of brain areas and structures that we know are affected by FTD. New techniques such as voxel-based morphometry can be used to obtain objective and quantitative measurement of gray and white matter, leading to detection of abnormalities in cortical size that cannot be seen by the usual visual inspection of the image. By using voxel-based morphometry and similar techniques for analyzing structural images, we may, in some cases, be able to detect brain changes before obvious clinical symptoms appear.

Although diseases like FTD are thought to be diseases of middle to old age, we don't know how early the disease process begins. For example, even though the majority of FTD patients have the onset of the symptoms that define their disease in their fifties, it may be that neuronal loss begins much earlier than that but the symptoms appear only after a certain proportion of brain tissue is damaged. Structural neuroimaging using voxel-based morphometry or similar techniques might be used to identify changes in brain tissues in asymptomatic patients at risk for developing FTD. This kind of study is best done with at-risk family members when a diagnosis of FTD occurs frequently within a family. A family history of FTD occurs in about a quarter of all patients who receive the diagnosis of FTD.

Functional neuroimaging (positron emission tomography [PET] or functional Magnetic Resonance Imaging [fMRI]) is a relatively new technology that allows scientists to see the brain at work based on energy consumption by neurons. These new techniques, for example, enable an estimation of the quantity of oxygen brain tissue is using or how much glucose is being utilized by specific regions of the brain. Doctors use functional neuroimaging in two ways. In one use, the patient is resting while doctors look at his brain activity. These "resting" scans can be quite helpful when an FTD patient with abnormal clinical symptoms characteristic of the disease has her structural brain imaging read as normal by an experienced neuroradiologist. It may be possible that functional imaging may reveal abnormal brain activity in FTD *prior* to changes to the structural anatomy of the brain.

Another use of functional neuroimaging is to study the brain activity of patients while they perform a cognitive task such as remembering a story or making a decision. When normal people perform these tasks while their brain activity is being recorded, their performance evokes a characteristic pattern of brain activity. When patients with brain disorders perform these same tasks, they often show changes in the pattern of brain activity that indicate they can no longer use some of the brain areas normally used to do the thinking required by the task. This observed change in the profile of brain activity in patients can sometimes help in the diagnosis of a brain disorder as well as help researchers understand how the brain reorganizes its functional capabilities after a disease begins to destroy a specific area. In the future, patients with a diagnosis of FTD will undergo functional neuroimaging as an important adjunct to their medical evaluation.

Patients with FTD usually are examined with neuropsychological testing as part of their diagnostic evaluation. The neuropsychological testing serves at least two purposes. One is to characterize the overall pattern of deficits in patients with FTD, to determine if a patient's individual findings fit into a subtype of FTD, and to recommend how to best manage the patient's symptoms. The second purpose is to identify the functions of the frontal and temporal lobes by studying people who have damage to those areas of the brain. The frontal lobes remain the most mysterious part of the human brain. Most researchers believe that this is the area of the brain that defines us as humans and differentiates us from other primates. The fact that patients with FTD most often have involvement of the frontal lobes of the brain means that we can learn about the normal functions of the frontal lobes by identifying what specific problems FTD patients have when it is damaged. Besides attaining a basic understanding of the functions of the frontal lobes, these studies will allow us to develop more sensitive and specific neuropsychological tests to evaluate the frontal lobes.

So what does the near future hold for clinical, biomedical, and basic scientific research on FTD? In the near future, clinical scientists need to develop consortiums to administer drug studies. Neuro-epidemiologic studies are very important and needed as they may identify risk factors for the development of FTD. Better methods to assay chemical concentrations in the brain via the spinal fluid, blood, and via functional neuroimaging are also needed. Identification of deficient neurotransmitter function in FTD can hasten proper drug applications for treating symptoms of FTD. Long-term goals include a better characterization of the molecular biology of the disease, the identification of genetic markers and environmental risk factors, and finally and crucially, targeted effective treatments to stop, reverse, or prevent the disease process.

Without an unexpected scientific breakthrough, we will be attempting to tackle the curing of FTD for the next few decades, since FTD receives relatively little government and private funding. On the other hand, other neurological disorders that receive a lot of public and private funding, like Alzheimer's disease and Parkinson's disease, are still not curable though there are some treatments available that can stabilize or improve symptoms for each disease.

The slow pace of this progress impacts on the family members of FTD patients in a number of different ways. On November 14, 2002, the Association for Frontotemporal Dementias was officially established. This association is desperately needed as a clearinghouse for new findings, as a support organization, as a lobbying organization, and for funding small grants and other initiatives. More specialized training for nursing home workers needs to include the description and management of FTD patients. Insurance companies and government agencies need to be have a better awareness of FTD and its unique symptoms so it is not lumped together with other dementias such as Alzheimer's disease. A small way in which you can help speed up research is by volunteering to participate in research studies on FTD at your local university or private medical center. This allows you to directly contribute to research. In the end, scientists and clinicians who want to cure FTD cannot advance easily without your direct involvement in research. In addition, you are encouraged to find ways to join or contribute to organizations that fund research on FTD. You must educate yourself to know as much about FTD as a nonspecialist can, so you can be an educated consumer of the medical care your loved one receives.

The future of biomedical research on FTD requires the interest and involvement of scientists and you. We are intertwined in this endeavor. When scientists make a new discovery they will seek your loved one's help by asking him to volunteer for research projects so that the scientists' ideas can be tested. Conversely, your involvement in the scientific process by encouraging more research on FTD will bring more funding and scientists to address the problem. It is this mix of family and science that will eventually lead to a cure for FTD.

Part II
Managing Daily Care

CHAPTER 10

Self-Expression and Safe Eating:

Understanding Speech, Swallowing, and Nutrition

ERICA WOLLMAN

This chapter discusses communication and swallowing and provides knowledge, experiences, and resources. Although most of these techniques work for most patients, they should not be substituted for professional care. Each person is unique and requires individualized attention. Therefore, working cooperatively with healthcare professionals, including a speech therapist or speech pathologist, is vital to optimum care.

COMMUNICATION

Communication is an essential part of life. It is not only how you express your needs and wants but also how you state your thoughts and novel ideas. It involves many different pathways to get a thought to materialize into expression. This is a concept that most people take for granted. However, you come to realize the complexities of communication when you encounter a person who has communication difficulties. The brain has many pathways that need to be utilized to get a thought from the brain to the mouth and tongue. If any of these pathways are disrupted, as they are in cases of FTD, then communication becomes impaired. Most people require guidance when it comes to communication. It is easier to make a choice when given only two options, and faces are full of expression. Nonverbal communication, such as facial expressions and gestures, is a way to help express yourself. Most of us talk with our hands as well as our voices and usually do not realize it. It is easy to complete people's sentences when we know the topic. For example, when given the stimulus phrase "up and _____," most people readily say "down." This is how brains are programmed. When given the stimulus phrase "open the _____," it is not as easy to fill in the blank. The answer could be "door, jar, window, book" and a number of other possibilities. This is why the phrasing of questions is so very important for people with degenerative neurological diseases.

Also, it is easier to communicate with people when the topic is a familiar one. Reminiscing is an excellent way to have a conversation. Use old pictures and talk about what you see, what you remember, and how you felt. Try not to bombard the person with questions. It is overwhelming to have multiple questions asked at one time. The goal is to have a conversation with a person. Fortunately, old memories stay with us for a longer time. Making a scrapbook with information and pictures is one way to stimulate conversation. Add pictures as time goes on, but try to keep the book uncomplicated.

Social conversation and singing are other ways to stimulate conversation. How many times has someone asked you, "How are you?" and the person responded with "I'm fine," before you even answered the question? This is an example of social language. It is an easy, light conversation where you can predict most of the conversation.

Unfortunately, with FTD, a person eventually is unable to talk because he loses the ability of the brain to coordinate speaking and send messages to the tongue and mouth to produce speech. Singing uses a different part of your brain and most people enjoy it even if all they can do is hum a few notes or mumble a tune.

STAGES OF QUESTIONS

Some questions are easier to answer than others. When you are given only two choices, it is easier to pick an answer. When given infinite choices, it requires more brainpower to figure out what you want. For example, the cook in the household is known to ask other family members, "What do you want for dinner?" and of course, the response is typically, "Anything." Most cooks at this point would respond, "I don't know how to make that!" It takes too much energy and thinking to go through all the possible choices you could have for dinner. When asked if you want pizza or hot dogs for dinner, you always answer with one of the choices. Soon you learn to give only two choices and the cook experiences less frustration and you get what you want for dinner.

Questions are very confusing. Sometimes you think you are asking a simple question when you are actually asking one with a world of possible answers. There are different levels of questioning that can be used as FTD progresses. To improve communication when the disease has progressed to a moderate level, ask questions that offer only two choices. For example, instead of asking, "What do you want to drink?" ask, "Do you want apple or grape juice?" When the disease becomes more severe, encourage communication by asking yes/no questions. At this point, it is becoming more difficult for the person to talk, and with this type of question you can still get a head nod as a response.

LEVELS OF QUESTIONING

As the disease progresses, it is important to change the way you ask questions to accommodate the thought processes of the person. There are three levels of questions that make answering easier as communication gets harder and as a person can no longer answer a simple question like, "How are you." The following chart shows examples of the way questions might be phrased as the disease progresses.

Mild speech problems	*Moderate speech problems*	*Severe speech problems*
What are you hungry for?	Do you want pizza or a cheeseburger?	Do you want a sandwich?
What do you want to drink?	Do you want apple or grape juice?	Do you want apple juice?
How are you?	Are you tired or hungry?	Does your head hurt?
Who is that?	Is that Mary or Jane?	Is that Mary?

Unfortunately, there is a point when the person suffering with FTD can no longer communicate. This is usually the hardest time for caregivers because you want to speak with the person. Touching the person's hand, forehead, or cheek continues to let him know you are there and that you care. Continue to talk to her even though she is not responding. Telling a story, reading the newspaper aloud, and reading books aloud are some ways to continue communication. Use the scrapbook you made to look at pictures.

In summary, caregivers can change the way a question is asked to help promote communication. The level of questioning will change as the disease progresses. Using scrapbooks, pictures, and reading can help make communicating an enjoyable experience.

UNDERSTANDING SWALLOWING

Most people believe swallowing is an easy thing to do, but actually it is one of the most complex activities that the body performs. Because it involves reflexes, muscles, and nerves working simultaneously, it is fascinating that people do it without much thought.

Swallowing begins with the eyes. How many times do you say, "That looks good," only to find out that it does not taste as good as it looks? When you see something you think is going to taste wonderful and you smell the aroma, your mouth starts to water. This excess saliva is required to help break down the food and help move it to the back of your mouth and down your throat.

Next, you open your mouth wide enough to get the food inside and begin to chew. Unfortunately, this is where some people get stuck. The person starts to chew and cannot get out of the chewing cycle and ends up constantly chewing. It is said that he "forgot to swallow." Actually, the person is stuck in the chewing cycle and his brain does not tell his tongue to swallow the food.

Once the food is chewed, then the tongue pulls it together into a ball (called a "bolus") and starts to push it to the back of the mouth. As this happens, you stop breathing, your throat elevates to close off your airway and open your esophagus, and the food bolus is pushed down the throat and into the esophagus. All of this happens in one second. As the food enters the esophagus, the throat relaxes and drops and you can now breathe. Now imagine how fast you pour a drink and how difficult it is to hold in your hands without a cup. Your mouth and throat have to try to control liquids every time you take a sip. Regular liquids are the most difficult texture to swallow, especially water. You have spots in the back of your throat that are sensitive to water and you will cough and choke if the water touches these spots when your throat is not elevated. Also, food and liquid follow the laws of physics. Yes, it is physics. When the tongue pushes the food down your throat, the bolus will go to the path of least resistance. Unfortunately, while you are breathing, the path of least resistance is your airway, and if you haven't closed off your airway fast enough, then the food or liquid will take that path. Your first reflex is to cough because coughing is the only way your body can clear the airway. If the cough is weak, then it usually sounds like clearing your throat. If the food or drink is not cleared out of your airway by coughing, it proceeds down into your lungs. Your lungs cannot digest food or liquid; therefore, it remains in your lungs. Your lungs then begin to produce mucus in hope that you will cough out the mucus along with the food or drink. This is the beginning of pneumonia and only takes two to four days to develop. Pneumonia usually recurs every three to six months if the swallowing problem is not corrected.

Signs of Aspiration or Pneumonia

If any of these symptoms occur, then it is recommended you call your doctor.
1. a spike in temperature while eating or shortly after eating
2. increased congestion
3. eyes watering and nose running while eating
4. difficulty breathing while eating and after eating

Safe Swallowing Techniques

There are several ways to help a person who is coughing or having difficulty with food and liquids. First, putting his chin to his chest and swallowing (called a "chin tuck") reduces the amount of muscle effort needed to close off his airway. It is usually recommended to use a straw and have the person tilt his head down to the straw to get his head into this chin tuck position. A person who has difficulty with straws can use one to three pillows behind his head to keep his head facing downward.

If this is difficult, then thickening the liquid can help. A thicker liquid swallows slower and may give the person the extra time needed to achieve airway closure. You can use an artificial thickener (like Thick It) or try making smoothies in the blender with yogurt or pudding.

When a person is not drinking regular liquids, it is important to keep her hydrated. Use snacks of ice cream, sherbet, pudding, yogurt, and creamy Popsicles during the day for hydration.

Levels of Liquid Swallowing Difficulties

Mild swallowing difficulties	Moderate swallowing difficulties	Severe swallowing difficulties
Drink regular liquids using chin tuck with a straw. May need to cut straw in half to create a shorter pathway for liquid.	Thicken liquids to nectar consistency (like milkshakes). May need to use chin tuck. Make smoothies in blender using yogurt.	Thicken liquids to honey/pudding consistency. May need to use spoon to eat it.

Changing Food Texture

In the early stages of a chewing problem, you can use a blender or knife to chop the food. You want pieces to be the size of a pea. In the later stages of a chewing problem, give the person a smooth-textured food like mashed potatoes to help "wash down" the food. You can also use a drink. Sometimes just telling the person to swallow works the best. If you notice that none of these techniques are working then it may be time for pureed foods. Purees are the easiest to swallow and require no chewing. Puree is the term for smooth foods; some foods in regular diets are considered pureed. Mashed potatoes, applesauce, and oatmeal are all examples of everyday foods that are considered pureed. Egg salad, casseroles, and tuna salad are soft foods. Again, you can use a blender to puree regular foods. Most foods are dry, so you will need to add a sauce or liquid into the blender to get the smooth texture. For pasta, you add the tomato sauce, then puree the pasta with the sauce. For meats, add gravy or some broth to achieve the smooth texture.

As the disease progresses, you will need to change the solid food textures to help with the person's chewing abilities.

Levels of Chewing Problems

Mild chewing problems	*Moderate chewing problems*	*Severe chewing problems*
Use extra gravy and sauces to help wash down food. Cut up meat to bite-size pieces and cook vegetables longer to make them soft.	Chop food in blender to make pea-size pieces. Use extra sauces and gravies to help wash down the food and keep it moist. May need to use canned vegetables and chop them into small pieces.	Using a blender, make food into a mashed potato texture (puree). Add sauce, gravy, or broth into blender with food to keep it smooth and moist.

Nutrition is important to keep a person healthy. If you are altering the food texture, you want to be sure she is eating enough calories and getting the needed nutrients. Talking with a registered dietitian is useful at this time. You can get a referral from your physician. The dietitian can recommend how many calories are needed and recommend nutritional supplements.

Swallowing difficulties can occur during any time as the disease progresses. It is important to maintain safe eating and drinking and consume the adequate amount of calories and nutrients. The speech therapist collaborates with the occupational therapist and nutritionist, who are specialists in eating and diet/caloric intake, respectively, to determine a comprehensive safe swallowing and easily fed diet.

ADMINISTERING MEDICATIONS

Taking medications becomes more problematic as a person's swallowing difficulty progresses. For pills, use applesauce, pudding, or yogurt to "wash it down" rather than liquids because the food does not dissolve the medication (which is meant to reduce the likelihood the meds will get stuck) and makes it easier to swallow. Give him an additional spoonful of applesauce, pudding, or yogurt (without medication) to clear his mouth of any remaining medication. If this continues to be difficult, it may be necessary to crush pills. You can buy a pill crusher at your local pharmacy. Mix the crushed pill with applesauce or pudding followed by an additional spoonful without medication to help wash it down.

For liquid medications, ask your physician if it can be changed into a solid medication. Or you can mix it with pudding or a thick liquid to help make it into a thicker texture. The patient can choke on liquid medications if he is having difficulty drinking regular liquids.

NEED A SPEECH PATHOLOGIST?

It is time to see a speech pathologist when any of the following occur:
- coughing constantly when eating
- food is held in mouth without swallowing
- significant weight loss (usually 5 to 8 percent of usual weight)
- pneumonia

The speech pathologist may recommend a fiber-optic endoscopic evaluation of swallowing (FEES) or a radiographic swallowing assessment done with a radiologist—known as a modified barium swallow. These types of studies allow visualization of the structures and allow the coordinated/uncoordinated swallowing mechanism to be viewed when an individual is fed samples of food of different consistencies (thin liquids, thick liquids, pureed solids, mechanical soft solids). Based on these data, safe food consistencies and specific compensatory strategies can be made by the speech therapist to maintain nutritional status by oral intake. These studies are quite effective in detecting "silent" aspirators, when swallowing difficulties are not realized during the clinical examination first performed by the speech pathologist. A barium swallowing study allows visualization of food/liquid passage through the esophagus and into the stomach. A barium swallow also allows assessment of an uncoordinated esophagus and reflux of gastric contents out of the stomach and into the esophagus and throat.

A FEEDING TUBE FOR NUTRITION AND HYDRATION

When safe swallowing is no longer possible, you should discuss a feeding tube with your doctor. This tube is inserted into the patient's stomach, and nutrients and medications are administered through this tube. At this point most people are thinking, "Don't let this happen to us." However, try to think of feeding tubes in a different way.

First, since the feeding tube allows a person to get proper nutrition, he may beome strong enough to eat little bites of some foods he enjoys. Second, the feeding tube allows medication, including pain medication, to be easily administered, enabling him to be as comfortable as possible. In addition, it may reduce the chance of contracting pneumonia.

There are several forms of nutrition and hydration:

1. *Peripheral intravenous feeding*—a vein in the arm receives intravenous fluids.
2. *Central intravenous feeding*—a catheter is inserted into a central vein near the heart to receive nourishment.
3. *Nasogastric tube*—a thin plastic tube is inserted through the nose and into the stomach.
4. *Gastrostomy tube*—a tube is surgically inserted through the abdominal wall into the stomach.
5. *Jejunostomy tube*—a feeding tube is inserted through the abdominal wall into the small intestine.

Ultimately, the decision to use a feeding tube is up to the caregiver or the patient through her advance directive. (see chapter 21 for more information.) The caregiver needs as much information as possible about benefits and problems or side effects. Educated decisions are the best decisions. Talk to your doctors, family members, friends, therapists, and whomever you can. The Internet has lots of information about advance directives, but be careful about what you find on the computer.

SUMMARY

FTD is a progressive disease that affects a person's communication and swallowing skills. Using scrapbooks, reminiscing, and singing are ways to continue to communicate. Also, swallowing can be made safer by thickening liquids and changing solid textures. Speech language pathologists and registered dietitians are available to help you throughout the progression and can provide you with helpful suggestions.

Definitions

Speech pathologist: a person with a degree and/or certification in speech and language pathology who is qualified to diagnose speech, language, swallowing, and voice disorders and to prescribe and implement therapeutic measures.

Modified barium swallow study: a radiographic study with a speech pathologist and radiologist designed to study the oral and pharyngeal stages of the swallow. The patient is given various food and liquid textures mixed with barium. Also known as videofluoroscopy, video swallow study, and cine esophagram.

Fiber-Optic Endoscopic Evaluation of Swallowing: a study that uses an endoscope inserted in the patient's nose and down his throat. The speech pathologist gives the person various liquid and food textures and watches the substances being swallowed. Also known as FEES.

Swallowing evaluation: a clinical evaluation with a speech pathologist where the person is given various food and liquids. The speech pathologist uses clinical judgment, observation of the person's management of the textures and observation of the person's response to the textures after several minutes.

RESOURCES

ASHA: American Speech and Hearing Association, 10801 Rockville Pike, Rockville, MD 20852, 800-498-2071, www.asha.org

Thick It: Precision Foods, Inc. (dry powder used for thickening foods and drinks), 800-333-0003, www.precisionfoods.com. (Available at local pharmacies.)

Simply Thick: Phagia-Gel Technologies, LLC (gel used for thickening foods and drinks), 1374 Clarkson Road, St. Louis, MO 63011, 800-205-7115, www.simplythick.com.

Bruce Medical Supplies (eating and drinking utensils), 411 Waverly Oaks Road, Suite 154, Waltham, MA 02452, 800-225-8446, www.brucemedical.com.

AliMed Inc. (makes pureed food, has feeding equipment), 297 High Street, Dedham, MA 02026, 800-225-2610, www.alimed.com, www.dysphagiatherapy.com.

Non-chew Cookbook by J. Randy Wilson, Wilson Publishing, Inc. 5708 Nicollet Ave. South, Minneapolis, MN 55419, 800-843-2409.

Martin, Janet and Jane Backhouse. *Goodlooking, Easy Swallowing Cookbook.* Woburn, Mass.: Butterworth-Heinemann, 1993.

CHAPTER 11

A Step Ahead:

Exercise and Mobility

HEATHER J. CIANCI

WHAT IS PHYSICAL THERAPY?

In the treatment of FTD, the role of rehabilitation is to preserve as best as possible the functional ability of the patient in everyday activities. Through the use of the therapies discussed in chapter 6, assistance can be provided to both the patient and caregiver throughout the entire disease process. Training and education in mobility and safety can help to lessen the challenges faced throughout the disease. This chapter will look at how physical therapy can help those with FTD.

Physical therapy is a rehabilitative service provided by physical therapists and physical therapists' assistants under the direction of a physician. Physical therapists evaluate patients' limitations by assessing their joints, muscles, mobility, balance, and activities of daily living. Once the therapist determines the cause of the limitation, the physician and therapist prepare a plan of care for treatment. The treatment plan can be followed through by a physical therapist or a physical therapist's assistant. Treatments can consist of strength and flexibility training, the learning of new mobility techniques, training with assistive devices such as walkers or wheelchairs, balance training, and aerobic conditioning. Physical therapy does not just deal with the patient's physical limitations, but also with the challenges the caregiver may face. Therapy can teach new ways to help caregivers safely assist their loved ones, new ways of setting up the home to prevent falls and other injuries, and new ways of helping those with FTD still participate in activities they enjoy.

RECEIVING PHYSICAL THERAPY

To receive physical therapy, a physician must write a prescription for the service, just as she would for medication. This is the case whether the patient is being treated in a hospital, outpatient facility, or at home. If the treatment is taking place in a hospital or at home, the therapist will come to the patient, having taken care of most of the insurance requirements beforehand. However, if the treatment is to take place in an outpatient facility, the responsibility of fulfilling the insurance requirements will fall to the caregiver. There even may be times when the responsibility of obtaining a prescription for physical therapy will also fall to the caregiver. Some physicians do not regularly deal with physical therapy, and the caregiver may need to request the service. As a caregiver, it is important to look for every opportunity available to help you and your loved one. Physical therapy can do just that.

DEALING WITH YOUR HEALTH INSURANCE PROVIDER

Once the prescription for outpatient physical therapy is obtained, you must review your health insurance requirements. Many HMOs will only allow services to be provided at certain facilities (this is referred to as being "capitated" to a facility) for a certain period of time. Others may require an insurance referral form to be completed by the physician in addition to the prescription. Even when capitated to certain facilities, you have the right to petition your insurance to go elsewhere. Although this may be time consuming, if your physician is willing to assist you, it is possible. There must be a valid reason for wanting to receive services at another facility. These reasons can include: the specialties of the therapy staff, a prior poor experience with the facility, distance, or the ratio of therapy staff to patient (those with dementia tend to perform better with one-on-one, consistent care).

Those with Medicare generally have an easier time receiving therapy. Medicare allows for visits at any facility and requires no referral forms. As with all insurances, visits are not unlimited. Once a patient reaches his goals, or stops showing signs of improvement, the therapy will be discontinued. For this reason, it is important to discuss the goals of treatment with the therapist as soon as care begins. Goals should be aimed at improving mobility techniques, preventing deconditioning and falls, and slowing functional decline as much as possible. All of these work together toward the greater goal of keeping the patient independent as long as possible.

FINDING THE RIGHT THERAPIST

Determining how far progressed your loved one is in her dementia will help to determine which therapist and/or facility is best. Those who are in the early stages may not require as much one-on-one attention as those who are more progressed. For those who are more progressed in their disease, it is recommended that they receive therapy by a therapist who is able to spend more one-on-one time during treatment. Outpatient facilities that primarily deal with the neurological or geriatric population tend to do well with providing this type of care. Calling ahead to find out the therapist-to-client ratio can assist with making this decision. You can also inquire about the therapy staff's experience in treating patients with dementia. Through the American Physical Therapy Association, you can receive information on therapists who are board-certified specialists. Again, you may want to look to those who specialize in neurology or gerontology. Above all, the most important things to look for in your therapist are compassion, the ability to communicate with you and your loved one, and the comfort level you have when you are together. A trusting relationship will help to foster good results.

THE PHYSICAL THERAPY PROGRAM

Common Physical and Functional Changes in Those with FTD

The degeneration of the brain that is seen in FTD can indirectly cause a degeneration in functional ability. The following table shows how the two can be related. By being aware of the potential injuries that can occur, you will be better prepared to help your loved one maintain physical well-being.

Frontotemporal Degeneration	*Physical/Functional Changes*
Loss of initiative and decreased interest in daily activities	Less movement, muscle weakness and atrophy, stiffness, risk of skin breakdown
Impaired judgment	Falls, burns, various injuries
Excessive manual exploration of the environment	Falls, burns, lacerations of hands
Decreased ability to read or write	Injuries from inability to recognize safety hazards
Apraxia—loss of skilled movement abilities	Muscle weakness and atrophy, stiffness, difficulty with self-care and walking, falls
Spatial neglect—inability to properly recognize body or objects to one side	Muscle weakness, stiffness, difficulty with self-care and walking
Increased muscle spasticity or tone	Muscle contractures, impaired mobility and posture, skin breakdown—decubitus ulcers/bed sores

Physical Therapy in the Beginning Stages— The Patient's Program

Beginning a course of physical therapy early after the diagnosis can have many benefits. At this stage, patients are the most likely to be able to learn and incorporate new movement techniques, exercises, and safety instructions into their everyday lives. Starting therapy early on will also help patients and families to establish a rapport with their therapist. Establishing an early relationship with a therapist can help to foster a smoother transition between the stages of change. This way, the therapist will better know the patient's history and needs each time it is necessary to restart physical therapy.

It is not uncommon for those diagnosed with FTD to suffer early on from some balance problems. You may notice that your loved one looks a little unsteady while walking, especially when turning. You may also notice that she has changed the way she normally performs tasks, such as getting out of bed or getting dressed. This is the time to begin outpatient physical therapy. A program can be started to work on balance, mobility techniques, and fall prevention. You should also be learning a home exercise program to help maintain muscle strength and joint flexibility. Remember, for a program to be fully effective, exercises must be performed at home, not just in the clinic.

Many exercises can be performed at home without using fancy equipment or machines. Therapists can give you Theraband, an elastic resistance band used to strengthen muscles. The corner of a room can help with stretching the pectoralis muscles, located in the front of the chest. This can be accomplished by simply placing the forearms and hands along each wall of the corner and then leaning the body through the arms. (See figure 1.)

A chair can be used to perform chair dips to strengthen the triceps muscles, located on the back of the upper arm. Simply sit on the edge of the chair and try to lift your bottom up off of the chair by using only your hands on the arm rests. (See figure 2.) A walk outside for at least fifteen minutes will work on circulation and endurance.

Some people prefer to continue their exercise program at home after the completion of formal physical therapy because of changes in their loved one's behavior (speech problems, disinhibition, etc.). There are those who choose to join or to continue at a gym for their exercise program. Care should be taken that your loved one is still safe using exercise equipment. You may wish to have a trainer assist with the exercise program or attend the gym with your loved one.

Aquatic therapy can be beneficial for those with FTD. Warm water soothes tight muscles and gives support to those with balance

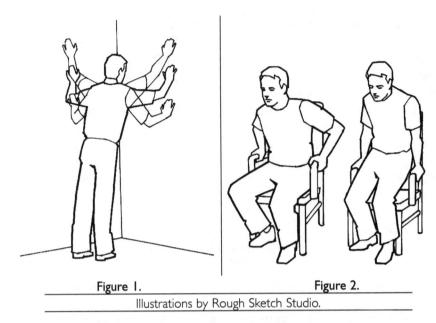

Figure 1.   Figure 2.

Illustrations by Rough Sketch Studio.

problems. Strength, endurance, and balance are just a few of the issues that can be addressed through an aquatic therapy program. This must be prescribed by a physician and overseen by a physical therapist. Local gyms may run group water exercise programs, but remember that these are mainly general exercise programs and are not aimed at individuals' specific needs.

Physical Therapy in the Middle Stages—
The Patient and Caregiver's Program

As people advance with FTD, they may begin to experience more difficulty with walking and mobility. Outpatient physical therapy can be used again to address these problems. Therapists can determine if an ambulatory assistive device, such as a walker, is needed. One type of walker that can be helpful is a four-wheeled rolling walker. This type of walker has brakes, a basket to hold belongings, and a seat. This type of walker is particularly helpful for those who still want to get out but may fatigue easily. The seat option means not having to also bring along a wheelchair and not always being on the lookout for chairs and benches. This type of walker is partially covered by most insurance with a prescription and letter of medical necessity from the physician. If walking outside or in unfamiliar places is becoming difficult, a manual wheelchair can be rented through the insurance carrier to make travel safer and easier. At this point, training for shower and bathtub transfers may also be necessary. Caregivers should be trained in how to safely manage themselves while helping their loved ones.

The home exercise program should continue, but now the caregiver may need to provide more assistance. Exercises should be revamped to address the particular needs of the patient at this stage. Rigidity may become more of a problem now, and exercises that emphasize stretching and rotational movements should be performed. Heating pads and massage to rigid areas may offer relief and work well in conjunction with exercise.

At this stage, balance may begin to become a problem. Once again, an ambulatory device can be helpful. Outpatient physical therapy may also need to restart. Through particular exercises, the therapist can work on "retraining" balance. However, if the balance itself cannot be improved, the environment always can. Placing handrails in the bathroom, moving furniture to open up space, and improving lighting can all improve safety. Education on how to prevent falls should always be included in the treatment plan. (See chapter 14 for more information.)

The therapist should also ensure that patients keep good posture. Learning about proper positioning while sitting helps to keep patients from slumping forward. This can improve breathing, swallowing, and decrease possible drooling.

One way to do this is to place a small towel roll along the lower back in the chair. This helps to keep the spine in a natural arch position with the shoulders and head upright.

If the patient cannot handle traveling to an outpatient facility, homecare therapy can be arranged. The therapist will work with the patient and caregiver within their own environment. Issues that are addressed in outpatient therapy can be addressed equally well in the home.

Physical Therapy in the Later Stages— The Caregiver's Program

As patients become less mobile, it becomes important to start addressing the prevention of skin breakdown. Sitting or lying in one position for even a few hours at a time can lead to skin breakdown. In addition, moisture from incontinence and/or perspiration can speed this process along.

Tissue that is over bony areas of the body, such as the elbows, heels, ankles, and sacrum, are commonly affected. Pressure to these areas from infrequent position changes leads to an impaired blood supply to that area. If not relieved, the skin can go from being red and irritated to ulcerated, eventually leading to muscle and bone death.

Those who are spending the majority of their time sitting should be reminded or helped to change their position every fifteen minutes. Those who are bedridden should be helped to change position every two hours. A specialized lift known as the Hoyer can be rented to help with transferring these patients in and out of bed for position changes. Most insurances will help to cover the cost of the lift.

Passive range-of-motion exercises performed by the caregiver can help with circulation and the prevention of contractures. Homecare therapy can teach caregivers how to perform these exercises for their loved ones. Instruction in proper positioning should also be taught by the homecare therapist. Specialized cushions, wedges, padding, and braces can be used in wheelchairs and beds to promote comfort and prevent contractures and skin breakdown. One example is a foot brace known as a pressure relief, ankle/foot orthosis (PRAFO). This brace helps to keep pressure off of the heel, while keeping the ankle in a position to prevent contractures. With a prescription from the physician, most of these items can be covered by insurance.

When a loved one can no longer safely ambulate, even with the use of an assistive device, a customized wheelchair should be considered. A wheelchair provides the patient with the ability to still have some functional independence, and makes mobility much easier and safer for the caregiver. Together, the therapist and physician will recommend which type of wheelchair is best for the patient. Generally, the wheelchair should be lightweight and have removable arm and leg rests. Along with this, a specialized pressure-relief cushion and seat belt should be included. Your loved one must be professionally measured to ensure the proper fit of the wheelchair. With a prescription and a letter of medical necessity from the physician, most insurances will provide coverage for wheelchairs. Some insurances will even help with the cost of ramps for the home. If your insurance carrier does not, be sure to check with your local agency of aging (AAA), support group, or a social worker recommended by your physician or therapist for suggestions on alternate funding.

PREVENTING FALLS

Fall prevention strategies should begin as soon as possible, due to the many factors that can contribute to falls. These factors are broken down into two categories: extrinsic and intrinsic. An extrinsic factor is something that occurs within the environment. An example would be slipping on a bathroom rug that does not properly grip the floor. Many extrinsic factors in the home can be modified rather simply and economically. The therapist can show you how to modify each room and which equipment will ensure optimal safety. (See chapter 14 for more information.)

An intrinsic factor is something that occurs within a person physically. An example would be falling due to dizziness from low blood pressure. A side effect of some medications is a rapid drop in blood pressure when moving from a sitting to standing position. Some common intrinsic factors in those with FTD are gait and balance changes, muscle weakness due to inactivity, and muscle rigidity/tightness. All of these changes can be helped to some degree through the use of physical therapy. Learning to use the proper assistive device with walking, building muscle tone through strengthening exercises, and reducing muscle tightness through stretching are all examples of how physical therapy can help reduce falls.

SUMMARY

Physical therapy provides many different treatment options to patients with FTD and their caregivers. Therapy can help to slow the progression of functional decline.

For this reason, it is important to get started in therapy as soon as functional changes occur. Because FTD is progressive in nature, many patients and caregivers feel a loss of control. However, by using treatments and equipment that focus on ability, rather than disability, physical therapy can give back some control to those affected by FTD.

BIBLIOGRAPHY

Berkow, R., and A. J. Fletcher, eds. *The Merck Manual,* 16th ed. Rahway, N. J.: Merck Research Laboratories, 1992.

"Family Caregiver Alliance fact sheet: Frontotemporal dementia" [online]. www.caregiver.org/factsheets/frontempC.html [January 16, 2002].

Guccione, A. "What is a physical therapist?" *American Physical Therapy Association* [online]. http://internet.apta.org/pt_magazine/oct99/closer.html [January 10, 2002].

Hodges, J. R. "Frontotemporal dementia (Pick's disease): Clinical features and assessment." *Neurology* 56 (2001): S6–S10.

Hutton, T. J. *Preventing Falls.* Amherst, N.Y.: Prometheus Books, 2000.

Perry, R. J., and B. L. Miller. "Behavior and treatment in frontotemporal dementia." *Neurology* 56 (2001): S46–S51.

"Pick's disease" [online]. http://health.yahoo.com/health/dc/ 000744/0.html [January 16, 2002].

Robinson, K. M. "Rehabilitation applications in caring for patients with Pick's disease and frontotemporal dementia." *Neurology* 56 (2001): S56–S58.

Rosen, H. J., et al. "Frontotemporal dementia." *Neurologic Clinics* 18, no. 4 (Nov. 2000): 979–92.

CHAPTER 12

Challenging the Mind:

Activities and Socialization

LISA ANN FAGAN

INTRODUCTION

Engaging in activities, or "doing things," benefits us in many ways. Activities can bring us joy or a sense of purpose. They can shape our identity and help structure our days and nights. Engaging in activities during the day can lead to more restful nights. Without meaningful activities and social roles, we would become so bored that time would seem endless, and we would have difficulty defining ourselves. One of the tragedies of dementia is that it alters a person's ability to participate in activities and relationships long before the body is ready to stop.[1]

FTD can cause a myriad of symptoms that can alter an individual's ability to engage in activities. Behavioral manifestations, including a decline in interpersonal conduct, poor impulse control, and depression, can cause social isolation and decreased opportunities for interaction.[2] Linguistic deficits common in FTD (word finding, word substitution, progressive nonfluent aphasia, semantic dementia, and other disorders) impact an individual's ability to communicate, thereby limiting social interaction.[3] Cognitive and perceptual changes, such as a decline in memory, inability to plan and sequence activities, and diminished visual-perceptual skills, can cause further limitations in initiating and participating in desired activities.[4]

A decline in active engagement with life (lack of activity participation and interpersonal relationships) has been linked to many negative outcomes, including depression, anxiety, pacing, and agitation.[5] Finding activities that are meaningful and provide successful experiences, and are not viewed as "childish" or "busy work," are a major challenge for caregivers.[6]

INDEPENDENCE ISSUES

Individuals with FTD are, first and foremost, adults. They have led successful lives, simultaneously balancing a variety of roles: spouse, parent, employee, hobbyist, religious participant, community volunteer, and others too varied to mention. Losing the ability to control one's own actions, thoughts, and feelings is distressing, and some individuals valiantly strive to remain autonomous in the early stages of dementia. In some individuals, there is an early loss of insight into their abilities, and the loss of self and abilities appears to cause them less concern than it does their family.

Activities and social interaction should promote maintenance of skills and abilities, compensate for declining capabilities, and incorporate familiar roles and routines of daily life. Allowing for choices in activities fosters a sense a control.[7] Success-oriented tasks allow the individual to feel pride in accomplishments, and sustain self-identity.[8]

THE JUST-RIGHT CHALLENGE— MODIFYING ACTIVITIES FOR SUCCESS

Finding the "just-right challenge" that balances abilities with interests is a daunting task for caregivers. To be able to complete a task independently, sometimes the activity must be simplified. Making cookies from a premeasured mix is easier than making them from scratch. Setting a table is easier if all the needed objects are gathered and put on the table before you ask the individual with FTD for assistance.

We often provide many directions for an activity at one time (e.g., "Finish watering the plants, then come inside and wash your hands before lunch"). Providing one-step directions may be needed to ensure successful task completion and promote continued independence (e.g., "Please water those plants" as you hand the individual a watering can, and point toward the plants that need attention). Many individuals find giving one-step direction challenging, but it gets easier with time and practice.

The environment in which the activity takes place can either promote independence or constrain abilities. Excess noise and excess clutter can cause difficulty in concentration, resulting in distraction from the desired task. An environment that is too hot or too cold can impact performance, as can an environment that is not well lit.

Your mood as a caregiver can influence the activity as well. If you are stressed or irritable, the individual with FTD may perceive your mood and become anxious as well. Anxiety often leads to decreased task performance. Try to remain calm, and maintain your sense of humor when possible.

SPECIFIC TYPES OF ACTIVITIES

Activities can be divided into four categories based on various characteristics of the tasks: activities of daily living, work/productive activities, play/leisure, rest/relaxation. These are the groupings used by occupational therapists to classify the intent of the activity.[9] These categories cover the range of activities and interactions in which an individual participates throughout the day. Individuals need a balance of these tasks to maintain a healthy lifestyle.

Activities of daily living (ADLs) include several tasks discussed in other chapters: grooming, hygiene, bathing, dressing (chapter 13), feeding (chapter 10), and mobility (chapter 11). Other ADLs include socialization, functional communication, and sexual expression. These activities promote physical and psychological health and well-being.

For many individuals with FTD, *socialization* is challenged by behavioral disinhibition that may not be understood by friends, neighbors, and distant relatives. It would be wise to discuss behavioral changes with visitors before the interaction, so that the visitor is not shocked or offended by comments made by the individual with FTD. Small gatherings (one to four individuals) are usually more successful than larger group activities.

Functional communication refers to the manner in which we express and receive information regarding thoughts, feelings, needs, and desires. Verbal language abilities, facial expressions, gestures and body language, written language, and use of symbols and pictures are all forms of functional communication. Individuals with FTD often have difficulty with verbal language and many have blunted affects, making it difficult to express emotions.

Occasionally, written language or symbols and pictures may provide a more accurate method of communicating than relying on verbal language and facial expression. For individuals with prior knowledge or experience with keyboards, typing may be more successful than oral communication. Picture boards (graphic depictions of commonly needed items, such as a glass of water, toilet, sweater, book, etc.) can be useful when an individual is unable to verbally request a specific item.

Sexual expression or engaging in intimacy is often severely altered by FTD. Individuals may make inappropriate comments or violate other social norms of conduct. Some may become apathetic to their partner's wants and needs, and seek only their own fulfillment. Others may become depressed and withdrawn, and will not initiate any forms of intimacy.

Work/productive activities include household tasks (meal preparation, cleaning, clothing care, money management, household maintenance, and other tasks), care of others (grandchildren, pets, etc.), and vocational and volunteer activities. These tasks can often be divided into chunks that can be easily managed by the individual with FTD, if the activity is meaningful and interests the person. These activities promote self-identity and self-esteem.

A gentleman who considers himself to be a good home maintainer might take pride in changing light bulbs, raking leaves, or balancing a checkbook. A woman who went to great lengths to keep the home neat might enjoy dusting or folding laundry. Meal preparation can be broken into many smaller activities: making a salad, setting the table, frosting a cake. Many individuals with dementia enjoy the unconditional love of pets. Feeding, grooming, petting, or walking an animal may be very rewarding activities.

The kitchen can present many safety hazards for individuals with dementia. If an individual is likely to attempt a cooking task involving the stove, an electrician can install a range cut-off switch. Chapter 14 provides more home safety recommendations.

Care must be exercised when deciding whether or not to let an individual with FTD baby-sit young children. Due to the difficulties with cognitive language and social skills that many individuals with FTD experience, another adult should always be present when young children are in the home.

Play/leisure activities are another source of meaningful engagement for many individuals. Amusement, spontaneous enjoyment, and self-expression are possible outcomes of play and leisure activities.[10] Although some previous pursuits may become too challenging as the disease progresses, many individuals are able to participate in some manner in former pastimes.

Games with complex rules (e.g., chess, Scrabble), may need to be played as a team, or in a simplified manner. Card games may need to be simplified from games with complicated rules (such as pinochle or poker) to simpler games (blackjack or matching games) to games of chance (such as war).

Physical activities (such as dancing or taking a walk) can provide exercise as well as recreation, as can playing catch with a grandchild.

Music is a terrific activity. For those who played the piano or other musical instruments, that ability often remains until late stages of dementia. Although they might not be able to read music or learn a new piece, many individuals have memorized musical pieces that they frequently played, and can still recall them. Others may simply enjoy listening.

Gardening is the most popular leisure activity in the United States. Many individuals enjoy puttering in the garden, pulling an occasional weed, cutting a few flowers, or picking a ripe tomato. Others enjoy tending to indoor plants (e.g., watering, removing dead leaves, repotting larger plants that have outgrown the present container). Gardening activities can provide links to the former self, and promote self-esteem.

Art can provide an outlet for many who are unable to express themselves verbally. Some individuals with dementia who previously thought of themselves as "unartistic" can produce beautiful, expressive works. Creating small pieces from modeling clay can be enjoyable for some. There are many colored plastic clay products available in art and craft stores. Others enjoy painting or coloring activities. Some individuals enjoy creating art from a blank canvas or paper; others benefit from the structure of adult-appropriate patterns books that they fill in with color. Pattern books cover a wide array of interests, from flowers and butterflies to trains, cars, and sport scenes. Patterns may be printed on translucent paper (creating a stained-glass effect) or on paper that accepts watercolors. One series of pattern books features outlines of famous works of art that you color or paint.

Reading is an activity enjoyed by many individuals. In the early stages of FTD, an individual might be able to read a large-print short story or poem aloud with a friend, family member, or caregiver, and discuss the story afterward. Others may enjoy hearing familiar poems or stories being read to them. Some people enjoy looking at or reading magazines. The photographs and shorter article length in most magazines are more easily understood than in bigger or longer publications.

Reminiscence activities, such as looking through photo albums or watching old family movies, may be a meaningful activity to some individuals. For others, it may cause confusion or sadness.

Family celebrations might be overwhelming for some individuals. Family members may not understand the behavior of the individual with FTD (see *socialization*), and the individual with FTD might not recognize friends and family or be able to verbalize names. Smaller groups tend to be easier to tolerate. Familiar traditions and rituals may need to be modified in response to the individual's capabilities (e.g., someone else might need to carve the Thanksgiving turkey or make the birthday cake).

Rest/relaxation includes passive activities (e.g., watching TV, listening to music) that require little participation, and spiritual activities that renew the soul. Some individuals have difficulty discriminating between TV and reality, and may become anxious when watching the news or action programs. Movies may be too long in duration for the individual to follow, but familiar movies might be enjoyed for brief periods. Avoid using children's programs as entertainment. There are several companies that make adult-appropriate videos (e.g., nature, animals, travelogs through foreign countries that the individual had visited). Some may be available at the local library.

Many individuals may not tolerate attending religious services, but enjoy televised or taped services, and familiar songs and hymns. Prayers learned in youth might be recalled and provide a source of comfort for some.

Some individuals benefit from stress reduction and relaxation techniques when anxious. A hand massage with scented lotion, some deep breathing exercises (with simple verbal cues, such as "Breathe in" and "Breathe out"), or reciting a favorite poem can assist a person to become calmer. Petting a cat or a soft-textured fabric (e.g., chenille or velvet) may work for other people. Finding an effective stress reduction or relaxation technique is an individualized process, but a very important one, if you are caring for a person who frequently becomes anxious. If the individual is unable to be calmed after several alternatives are attempted, the physician should be contacted.

EXERCISE

Daily physical activity is important for everyone, regardless of current fitness level.[11] Walking, dancing, swimming, riding a stationary bike, or other movement is recommended to maintain muscle mass, promote cardiovascular health, maintain flexibility and balance, decrease depression, enhance cognitive functioning, and promote general psychological well-being. For optimal cardiovascular benefit, aerobic activity is usually recommended for at least twenty minutes per session, three to five sessions per week, after approval from your physician. This topic is covered in more detail in chapter 11.

For some individuals, exercise can be made more enjoyable with music, videos, or as a game. Dancing or marching to favorite music, participating along with a video, playing basketball or golf, or imitating movements done by a caregiver are all forms of exercise.

Some individuals prefer a more regimented exercise program that includes hand-held weights, exercise bands, or pulleys. There are many styles of hand-held weights and cuff-style ankle/wrist weights available at sporting goods stores and mass-merchandise stores. Exercise bands are available at some sporting goods as well as through therapy supply vendors listed in the Resources. Over-the-door pulleys encourage full arm movement. They can be used as needed, then removed from the doorframe. They are available through the therapy supply vendors in the Resources.

FREEDOM AND SAFETY

Some individuals with dementia are at a high risk for wandering and/or getting lost, due to decreased topographical orientation (the ability to find one's way). Even familiar routes may become confusing at some point during the disease process. An individual may not be able to state where she lives or be able to give her name. Such an individual should wear an identification bracelet or necklace, so that police and rescue authorities could return a lost individual to his home. The Alzheimer's Association Safe Return program offers such an identification bracelet or necklace, along with a communications network to alert authorities of a missing person.

Home safety modifications are a vital part of a safety program. If possible, an enclosed yard offers a safe area to enjoy nature without the risks of wandering. See chapter 14 for more information.

DRIVING

For many individuals (with or without dementia), surrendering a driver's license is one of the most emotionally upsetting times in their life. Many individuals in the United States fear losing their driver's license more than death or going to a nursing home.[12] In the United States, being able to drive a car fosters independence and freedom.

In some states, a person cannot hold a driver's license once a diagnosis of dementia is made. In other states, there is no such restriction. A driving evaluation may be recommended by the neurologist or physician to determine if the individual is still capable of driving.[13] The evaluation is usually completed by an occupational therapist, and the results are sent to the referring physician and (if required by state law) to the Department of Motor Vehicles.

Individuals may still attempt to drive after a driver's license has been surrendered. In some cases, keys need to be hidden or cars need to be sold, so that the individual with dementia will not drive.

SUMMARY

Activities are the everyday tasks that provide our lives with meaning, shape our identity, and allow us to accomplish our daily routines. Dementia can rob a person of the ability to initiate a task or complete a complex activity. Tasks can be simplified, or given in one-step directions, to promote continued independence and success.

There are many types of activities, including activities of daily living, work/productive activities, play/leisure, and rest/relaxation. Activities that require special consideration include driving, babysitting, and other safety-related issues. Maintaining a balance of activities that are success-oriented and meaningful to the individual helps promote physical and psychological well-being.

TABLE I. The Do's and Don'ts of Activities Planning for Individuals with FTD
(adapted from *Activity Programming for Persons with Dementia: A Sourcebook*)

DO	DON'T
Treat the person as an adult	Speak to the person as if he/she is a child
Provide a calm environment	Yell at or scold the person
Simplify instructions	Give up
Establish a familiar routine	
Provide encouragement	
Be patient and flexible	
Help the person remain as independent as possible	

TABLE 2. Suggested Activities	
Exercise/Physical activity	Taking a walk Dancing Raking leaves/gardening Vacuuming Exercising (may need to follow demonstrated exercises)
Creative activities	Doing art projects (clay, painting, coloring) Playing musical instruments
Relaxation	Listening to music Watching TV or movies Getting a hand massage Singing religious hymns or saying prayers Petting a cat or dog
Cognitive stimulation	Listening to stories/poems Playing simplified word or card games Reminiscing (recalling family events)
Purposeful activities	Assisting with household chores (setting the table, folding laundry, etc.) Assisting with meal preparation Providing self-care (bathing, dressing, grooming) Giving pet care

RESOURCES

Exercise equipment is available from several vendors. An Internet search using the keywords "Theraband" or "over door pulleys" will yield several results. These are given as a sample of vendor sites.

Theraband, KAS Enterprises, 1317 W. 23rd Avenue, Covington, LA 70433, 877-860-9534 (toll-free), www.kasenterprises.com/theraband.

Over the Door Pulleys, PrePak Prdoucts, 4055 Oceanside Boulevard Ste L., Oceanside, CA 92056-5821, 800-544-7527 (toll-free), www.prepakproducts.com.

NOTES

1. J. M. Zgola, *Doing Things: A Guide to Programming Activities for Persons with Alzheimer's Disease and Related Disorders* (Baltimore: Johns Hopkins University Press, 1987); Alzheimer's Association, *Activity Programming for Persons with Dementia: A Sourcebook* (Chicago: Alzheimer's Association, 1995).

2. P. Mychack et al., "The influence of right frontotemproal dysfunction on social behavior in frontotemporal dementia," *Neurology* 56, no. 11, suppl. 4 (2001): S11–S15.

3. M. Grossman, "A multidisciplinary approach to Pick's disease and frontotemporal dementia," *Neurology* 56, no. 11, suppl. 4 (2001): S1–S2.

4. Ibid.; K. M. Robinson, "Rehabilitation applications in caring for patients with Pick's disease and frontotemporal dementias," *Neurology* 56 no. 11, suppl. 4 (2001): S56–S58.

5. J. W. Rowe and R. L. Kahn, "Successful aging," in *Healthy Aging: Challenges and Solutions*, ed. K. Dychtwald (Gaithersburg, Md.: Aspen, 1999); Zgola, *Doing Things*.

6. C. J. Camp, ed., *Montessori-based Activities for Persons with Dementia*, vol. 1 (Beachwood, Ohio: Menorah Park Center for Senior Living, 1999).

7. S. H. Briller et al., "Maximizing cognitive and functional abilities," in *Creating Successful Dementia Care Settings*, ed. M. P. Calkins (Baltimore: Health Professions Press, 2001).

8. Zgola, *Doing Things*; Alzheimer's Association, *Activity Programming for Persons with Dementia*.

9. American Occupational Therapy Association, *Occupational Therapy Practice Guidelines for Adults with Dementia* (Bethesda, Md.: American Occupational Therapy Association, 1999).

10. J. A. Brackley, *Creating Moments of Joy for the Person with Alzheimer's or Dementia* (Polk City, Iowa: Enhanced Living, 1999); American Occupa-

tional Therapy Association, *Occupational Therapy Practice Guidelines for Adults with Dementia.*

11. President's Council on Physical Fitness and Sports Research Digest, *Physical Activity and Aging: Implications for Health and Quality of Life*, series 3, no. 4 (Washington, D.C.: President's Council on Physical Fitness, 1998).

12. J. Diffendal, "Giving up the car keys: When are dementia patients unfit to drive?" *Advance for Occupational Therapy Practitioners* (17 July 2000).

13. Association for Driver Rehabilitation Specialists, *Fact Sheet on Driving and Alzheimer's/Dementia* (Edgerton, Wisc.: Association for Driver Rehabilitation Specialists, n.d.).

CHAPTER 13

Fostering Personal Care:
Hygiene, Dressing, and Eating

LISA ANN FAGAN

For individuals with a progressive neurodegenerative disease such as FTD, the ability to maintain maximal independence in the everyday activities of personal care (such as hygiene and dressing), or the ability of others to provide such care, becomes of paramount importance. Improvements in self-care tasks are not expected. However, the ability to maintain current levels of function is facilitated through strategies to reduce the effort required to achieve tasks, or by changing the environment to promote independence. A focus on assisting the individual by doing the personal care tasks *with* the person, instead of doing it *for* the person, is the key to maximizing remaining skills, and preventing overdependence on caregivers.

Another critical issue for individuals with FTD and their families is the maintenance of personal safety. In many individuals with dementia, their ability to conduct themselves in a safe manner is lost early in the disease process due to a number of factors, from sensory changes to impulsive behavior. Strategies for maintaining a safe environment for personal care will be discussed.

FACTORS AFFECTING ABILITY TO PARTICIPATE IN PERSONAL CARE

Psychosocial/Emotional Factors
- disinhibition of social norms (doesn't care what others think)
- depression (poor motivation to engage in any activities)
- fear of falling during personal care activities (limits willingness to move)
- paranoia, embarrassment, or anger

Cognitive Factors
- limited attention span (doesn't remember to complete all steps of an activity)
- decreased awareness of environmental cues (doesn't notice toothbrush in bathroom, forgets to brush teeth before bed)
- difficulty following complex verbal directions
- sequencing difficulty (can't figure out which item to put on first)
- perceptual deficits (puts right arm in left sleeve of a shirt)

Sensory Factors
- doesn't respond to internal cues (need to void, hunger/thirst/fullness, etc.)
- becomes distracted by background noises
- perceives touch as threatening

Physical Factors
- unable to plan body movements (difficulty putting leg in trousers)
- balance or mobility problems (difficulty standing or sitting without support)
- decreased coordination (difficulty fastening buttons)
- decreased endurance or strength from disuse (too tired to assist)

(Adapted from Hellen, 1998)

STRATEGIES TO ASSIST INDIVIDUALS WITH PERSONAL CARE TASKS

1. *Timing*—know when the individual is best able to assist (showers or baths might be more successful in the evening as opposed to the morning, or vice versa).

2. *Consistency*—a familiar caregiver, following a set routine, is often the most successful arrangement.

3. *Focus on abilities*—involve the individual in assisting as much as possible, and praise attempts (whether successful or not).

4. *Cueing*—give one-step directions ("Wash your face" as you hand the individual a washcloth)

5. *Distraction*—use singing, food, holding an item, etc. if the individual becomes upset during personal care activities, or to prevent the person from becoming upset.

6. *Mirroring*—an individual may be able to copy actions demonstrated by the caregiver (such as brushing teeth, combing hair, etc.).

7. *Chaining*—the caregiver initiates the activity, then the individual completes the task (such as buttoning, washing an arm or leg in the shower, shaving with an electric razor, etc.).

(Adapted from Hellen, 1998)

HYGIENE (Grooming, Toileting, and Bathing)

The ability to maintain body cleanliness, as well as complete activities related to elimination of body waste, is important for health and for social acceptance. While cultural norms may dictate higher or lower expectations of cleanliness, basic hygiene is important to prevent odors, infection, and disease. Individuals with dementia may not recognize the need for maintaining good hygiene due to disinhibition of social norms and other psychosocial and emotional factors, decreased sensory awareness, or decreased cognitive skills, as mentioned in the previous section.

Grooming includes the tasks we perform to maintain our appearance and health. These include activities such as brushing teeth and/or denture care; shaving; hair care; nail care; eye care (including applying glasses or contact lenses); ear care (including applying hearing aids); applying deodorant, powders, or lotions; and applying cosmetics.

In the early stages of FTD, environmental strategies such as leaving grooming items in a visible location alongside the sink may cue individuals to use the objects and complete tasks. For some, a daily checklist is helpful, to provide order and organization to the grooming routine.

In later stages, mirroring (demonstrating the tasks) is an effective strategy, as is chaining (initiating the task, and letting the individual complete the activity). Limiting the environmental cues can be helpful, because too many visible items can cause confusion.

In late stages, assistance from the caregiver is required. Allowing the individual to complete whatever steps of the grooming task they can is important to promote feelings of accomplishment, and to prevent overdependence on caregivers.

Toileting includes activities related to excretory body functions. Activities include clothing management, managing continence needs (including catheters or colostomies), cleaning the body, and applying protective equipment (such as disposable pads or briefs).

In early stages, environmental strategies, such as leaving the bathroom door open, may prompt the individual to use the toilet. Other environmental strategies include painting the wall behind the toilet a contrasting color to increase the visibility of the toilet, or installing a floor surface (linoleum, vinyl tile, carpeting) in a contrasting color. Another strategy is to mark a pathway with colored tape on the floor between the bed or chair, etc. and the bathroom, so the individual can follow the trail.

Verbal prompts on a regular basis (before or after meals, for example) can promote continued continence. Clothing that is easier to manage (such as elastic waist pants instead of zippered trousers) may allow for continued success with toileting.

In the later stages, more environmental modifications may be needed, including grab bars along the toilet to provide stability during transfers, and a raised toilet seat to make transfers easier for the caregiver.

If getting in and out of the bathroom becomes a challenge due to difficulty with transfers or mobility, a commode may be needed. Commodes can be rented or purchased from medical supply companies. Commodes come in several different styles, some with armrests that can be removed for sliding transfers (see page 190).

In the late stages, the individual may not respond to internal cues to void. Incontinence care may need to be provided, and disposable briefs may be used to avoid accidental soiling of clothing. While the individual is in bed, some caregivers use protective devices to prevent soiling of the bedding. Disposable absorbent pads can be placed on top of the fitted sheet, beneath the individual, and changed as need. Other caregivers prefer to use waterproof mattress pads.

Bathing includes cleansing of body parts (whether in a shower or tub, or by sink, or through use of newer products such as pre-moistened towelettes) as well as the rinsing and drying of the body. Many individuals with dementia have an aversion to bathing. The reason behind this phenomenon is not fully understood, but could be related to several factors:

- fear of water
- modesty
- fear of falling

Whatever the cause of the anxiety, assisting with bathing is one of the most challenging of all personal care tasks for the caregiver, and can be a significant factor in considering the need for professional assistance in the home or facility-based care.

Whatever method of bathing is selected, start by assembling all the necessary items: soap, shampoo or shower cap, washcloth, towels, robe, and any other products needed. You may want to wear a water-resistant apron or bathing suit to avoid getting your clothes wet. Make sure you have everything gathered; some individuals should not be left in the bathtub or shower alone while you get missing supplies.

Some individuals may be more calm during the bathing routine if soft music is playing, or if scented bath products are used. Others dislike being cold, and respond best in a warmer ambient temperature. A ceiling-mounted heat lamp may be helpful.

For all methods of bathing, the individual should be encouraged to assist as much as possible, from washing body parts after verbal or visual cues to completing the action once initiated by the caregiver.

For individuals who prefer taking a bath, getting in and out of the tub may be the most difficult and dangerous part of the task. Nonskid strips, decals, or a mat decrease the risk of slips or falls. A hydraulic or mechanical seat that raises and lowers the individual in the tub can be extremely helpful for the caregiver. There are models of bathtubs in which the side wall rolls down to allow the individual to easily enter and exit the tub. These tubs would replace the existing tub, but fit in the same space.

For assisting individuals who stand while showering, most caregivers report that using a stall shower is an easier option than showering in a bathtub. As with the bathtub, a nonskid floor surface will reduce the risk of slips and falls. Grab bars should be installed in and around the shower stall. They are important wherever the individual would reach for support when entering and exiting the shower stall, and where he would require support while standing during the shower. Grab bars can be installed vertically, horizontally, or on a diagonal, depending on need. An occupational therapist can assist in determining the proper location for grab bars. (See chapter 14 for further details regarding environmental modifications).

Many individuals are less fearful if they face away from the shower stream, facing the rear wall of the stall. A horizontally mounted grab bar on the rear wall can give the individual something to hold onto, for an increased feeling of support. A handheld shower is highly recommended by many caregivers, using the following strategies:

- Adjust the water temperature before directing water toward the individual.
- Use a gentle stream or mist of water.
- Start with a less sensitive part of the body, such as the feet.
- Move the water around the individual, instead of having the individual move.

(Adapted from Olsen, 1993)

For individuals who have difficulty standing, a bath or tub seat may be used. There are several styles from which to choose. A seat with a backrest is almost always preferable to a stool, as it provides more support. Other design factors to consider include armrests, seats that extend over the rim of the tub (to allow an individual to slide over the side of the tub, rather than step in and out of the tub), and padding. The individual's need for support and the available space in the bathroom may influence the decision to choose a style with or without armrests and/or an extended seat.

For individuals who are unable or unwilling to take a shower or bath, thorough cleansing can be accomplished by a sink or sponge bath, or by the use of commercially available premoistened towelettes. Dry shampoo (a powder that is applied to the head and brushed out) can be used if the individual does not like to have his hair washed.

DRESSING

We often dress in a manner that expresses our personal taste and style. For some individuals with dementia, maintaining the same style of dress as before the illness may be important to self-image and self-esteem. A former businessman may prefer to wear a shirt and tie every day; some ladies are accustomed to wearing a dress, jewelry, and make-up at all times. For others, clothing has little personal value.

We often take for granted the complex physical and cognitive skills involved in selecting and donning apparel. Choosing clothing from a full closet or dresser that is appropriate for the weather and which coordinates can be a daunting task for anyone. Limiting choices can be one strategy to simplify dressing. One way to limit choices is by keeping only seasonal items in the closet or hanging complete outfits on one hanger (pants/skirt and shirt/blouse) and letting the individual choose the outfit for the day. Another way to limit choices is by giving the choice between two items when ready to dress ("Do you want to wear the tan pants or the blue pants today?").

Some individuals prefer to wear the same outfit repeatedly, giving the caregiver little opportunity to clean the clothes. Buying multiples of the same outfit allows the caregiver to wash one set while the other is being worn.

Loose-fitting styles of clothing (such as elastic-waist pants in knit materials) and button-front shirts and sweaters are easier to put on than other styles. Shoes with hook and loop closures may be easier than tying laces. Shoes should have a rubber, non-skid sole and offer stability while walking and transferring.

Some individuals, when faced at one time with all items to be worn (undergarments, clothing, sweater, etc.) have difficulty determining which items to put on first. The proper sequence or order of which item goes on first is not recalled, and pieces of clothing can be skipped or put on top of other items (such as undergarments over pants or shirts). Layering clothing in the order in which it is put on is helpful in preventing such mistakes.

Some individuals need assistance only in starting the process of putting on an item of clothing. After the initial step (such as putting a sleeve into a shirt), they can complete the rest of the task.

Some individuals with FTD may undress themselves at socially inappropriate times. Clothing that is more difficult to remove, such as shirts that have buttons or zippers in the back, may be harder to remove, and consequently remain on longer. Avoid putting button-front shirts on backward, as they do not fit correctly and are uncomfortable. Other strategies to prevent disrobing include wearing multiple layers of clothing (e.g., undershirt, shirt, and sweater or vest), wearing clothing that is more challenging to remove (such as overalls or jumpsuits), and facing belt buckles toward the back instead of the front of the body.

EATING

We eat for a variety of reasons: to satisfy our hunger, to provide pleasure through our senses of smell and taste, to be polite in certain situations, and several other factors. Individuals with FTD often experience changes in habits and behaviors relating to food. They may overeat or constantly crave certain food items (especially sweets). They may disregard manners and social graces while eating, and may try to eat nonfood items.

To curb overeating, some caregivers limit access to the refrigerator or snack drawers through the use of locks on these areas, or they block access to the kitchen. While this may work for a brief period, many caregivers report that their loved ones find ways to obtain food regardless of the method used to prevent access.

To slow the pace at which some individuals consume food, weighted utensils may be used. The added resistance may slow the rate of speed with which they eat.

To reduce the likelihood that individuals may try to help themselves to food from someone else's plate, try using colored tape to mark a zone for each person at the table.

For individuals experiencing difficulty using utensils, a plate guard may be helpful. The device enables the individual to load food onto the utensil by pushing it against the plate guard and onto the fork or spoon. If the plate slides away from the individual, try using a nonskid placemat.

For individuals having difficulty holding cups, a mug may be easier to hold. Unbreakable cups and mugs should be used when possible. A bendable straw can also be used if drinking from a cup or mug becomes compromised.

When utensil usage becomes too challenging, an individual may still be capable of feeding themselves "finger foods." Fish sticks, chicken fingers, sandwiches, fruit and cereal bars, hard-boiled eggs, and tacos are all fingers foods, but there are many other possibilities as well. Almost any cooked meat can be wrapped in a flour tortilla; a scoop of tuna salad can be put on an ice cream cone. Many foods, while not necessarily neat, can be eaten by hand, including pieces of meatloaf, sausage links, waffles with jelly instead of syrup, and many others. These are but a few examples—use your creativity to think of other options.

SAFETY

Individuals with FTD often have difficulty with self-regulation and safety awareness. They may not realize the potential danger of situations, including cooking, using tools, smoking, and other activities.

Some caregivers have a cut-off switch installed on the stove or oven, so that the individual with FTD cannot turn on the range without supervision.

For individuals who use power tools, lawnmowers, and other tools, the basement or garage may need to be locked to prevent unsupervised access to these items.

If the individual smokes cigarettes, cigars, or pipes, they may need supervision or assistance with using matches or lighters.

Gentlemen may need supervision while shaving, and a safety razor or electric shaver should be used.

A lack of attention to sensory cues (such as water temperature in the shower) can lead to accidental scalding. Reducing the temperature setting on the hot water heater can prevent burns.

ASSISTING WITH TRANSFERS

In later stages of the disease, individuals may experience limitations in movement. They may require assistance getting up and down from the bed, chair, or toilet, and may need to use a wheelchair. Caregivers must be careful to avoid injuring themselves and the individual needing assistance, during transfers. There are a few basic safety points when assisting with any transfer:

- Make sure each person has nonskid footwear, securely fastened.
- Remember to keep your back as straight as possible—bend from the knees!
- Have the individual "scoot" forward toward the end of the seat.
- Make sure the individual's feet are on the floor, with heels slightly behind the front of the seat if possible.
- Have the individual lean slightly forward and place hands on armrests if available, or on the surface of the seat.
- Prepare the individual to stand (count to three, or give a short direction, such as "Stand up").
- Assist the individual as needed, either from the side (with a hand at or slightly below the waist, or under the arm), or from the front (with hands slightly below the waist). Do not pull the individual up by the arms.
- If you need to lift the individual, a transfer belt may be used.

(Adapted from Zgola, 1987)

A physical therapist or occupational therapist can teach you the proper method to assist with transfers so both you and your loved one are safe.

SUMMARY

Assisting individuals to maintain as much independence as possible in self-care tasks is an important part of caregiving. An emphasis on doing "with," rather than doing "for," the individual maintains dignity and self-esteem. Simplify activities to allow for continued participation by the individual with FTD, and modify tasks to ensure safety. As each person in the world is unique, so too is each individual with FTD. Not every strategy presented here will be helpful for each person; these are but a guide.

BIBLIOGRAPHY

American Occupational Therapy Association. *Occupational Therapy Practice Guidelines for Adults with Dementia.* Bethesda, Md.: American Occupational Therapy Association, 1999.

Briller, S. H., et al. "Maximizing cognitive and functional abilities." In *Creating Successful Dementia Care Settings*, edited by M. P. Calkins, Baltimore, Md.: Health Professions Press, 2001.

Hellen, C. R. *Alzheimer's Disease: Activity-focused care,* 2d ed. Boston, Mass.: Butterworth-Heinemann, 1998.

Mychack, P., et al. "The influence of right frontotemporal dysfunction on social behavior in frontotemporal dementia." *Neurology* 56, no. 11, suppl. 4 (2001): S11–S15.

Olsen, R. V., E. Ehrenkrantz, and B. Hutchings. *Homes That Help: Advice from Caregivers for Creating a Supportive Home.* Newark, N.J.: NJIT Press, 1993.

Perrin, T., and H. May. *Well-being in Dementia: An Occupational Approach for Therapists and Carers.* Edinburgh, Scotland: Churchill Livingstone, 2000.

Robinson, K. M. "Rehabilitation applications in caring for patients with Pick's disease and frontotemporal dementias." *Neurology* 56, no. 11, suppl. 4 (2001): S56–S58.

Zgola, J. M. *Doing Things: A Guide to Programming Activities for Persons with Alzheimer's Disease and Related Disorders.* Baltimore, Md.: Johns Hopkins University Press, 1987.

CHAPTER 14

Within These Walls:

Creating a Safe and Supportive Environment

LISA ANN FAGAN

According to interior designer Betsy Brawley, who specializes in designing environments for individuals with dementia, the environment is a "silent partner in caregiving."[1] A well-planned environment can be supportive and promote continued abilities and participation in activities, while a nonsupportive environment can lead to falls, agitation, and a decline in functional skills by limiting opportunities to participate in activities. This chapter will provide an overview of the role of the environment in supporting care, and strategies to improve the fit between the individual with FTD and his environment.

Just as no two persons are alike, no two environments are alike. The physical space, the objects in the space, and the interactions of the people in the space make each environment unique. The strategies presented in this chapter are ones that have worked for many individuals but may not be applicable or helpful in all situations. If there is a specific environmental challenge in your home, an occupational therapy home evaluation may be useful to determine an individualized environmental modification plan.

The need for environmental modification will change over the course of the illness, as well as in response to the aging process or other medical conditions the individual with FTD experiences. In the early stages of the disease, only minor modifications may be needed to simplify the environment and promote safety. As the dis-

193

ease progresses, more substantial adaptations may be needed, including installing grab bars, or making the home wheelchair accessible. Planning ahead is crucial. If you anticipate needing to make major changes (such as adding a first-floor bedroom or bathroom), it is best to start renovations when the individual is in the earlier stages of dementia. This gives her more time to adjust to the environment before she experiences further declines and is less able to adapt to changes.

CREATING A CALM AND REASSURING ENVIRONMENT

For many caregivers, creating a calming environment to reduce anxious or agitated behavior is the first goal of environmental modifications.[2] Various objects in the environment can frighten or upset the individual with dementia. Sensory overstimulation can also lead to anxiety. When the individual with dementia becomes stressed, he is unable to change the environment to reduce the source of the stress. He may try to escape the environment (wander away or attempt to leave the house), become combative or resistive during care, or have a catastrophic reaction. Eliminating the sources of environmental stress can reduce anxiety and promote a calmer atmosphere.

The following can be sources of environmental stress for some individuals. Suggested strategies to reduce the stress follow in italics.

Mirrors	The individual may not recognize her own reflection and be frightened that a stranger is in the house.
	—*Remove the mirror, or cover with a pull-down shade.*
Photographs	Some individuals do not recognize current pictures of friends and family members and are confused by them.
	—*Label the photographs, or remove the pictures and replace with photographs the individual recognizes (pictures taken during the years before the onset of the disease).*

Television	The individual may think there are other people in the room or may not be able to differentiate between reality and the television program.

—Do not watch violent or scary programs.
—Try nature programs, reruns of favorite shows, or old movies.

Excess noise	Too many sources of overlapping noise, such as the television, a barking dog, a ringing telephone, and a radio being played in a nearby room can cause auditory overstimulation.

—Reduce noise levels throughout the house. Use sound-absorbent materials (carpeting, drapes) to reduce noise levels.

Excess Glare	Unfiltered sunlight shining through windows or reflecting off of shiny surfaces, such as floors or mirrors, can cause visual stress.

—Use light-filtering window coverings (sheers, blinds, or shades).
—Consider nonglare floor surfaces (carpet, tile).
—Move mirrors that reflect sunlight.

Too little light, Uneven light levels	Shadows or dark areas within a room may cause fear.

—Provide increased lighting that covers a room with even levels of light.

Clutter	Too many objects in the environment can overstimulate.

—Reduce the number of items in the room.

Room temperature	Increased agitation has been reported in environments that were perceived as too cold or too hot by the individual.

—Regulate room temperature or add/remove a sweater as needed.

Seeing an area they can not access	Seeing the front yard or back deck but not being able to get there because the doors are locked can cause stress.

—Provide access to safe areas (fenced back yard) if possible.
—Cover windows to reduce distractions.

Locked doors   Some individuals are frustrated because they
                    want to be able to open the door and cannot do so.
                    —*Camouflage the door (paint or wallpaper the
                    door the same as the rest of the wall)*.

Unable to find   Some individuals are unable to remember
the bathroom   where the bathroom is located.
                    —*Keep the bathroom door open*.
                    —*Paint the bathroom door a different color than
                    the other doors in the house*.
                    —*Label the door with a sign that states "Bath-
                    room" or "Toilet" or with a picture of a toilet*.

For some individuals, creating an environment that includes pleas-
urable sensory experiences can be calming. The following strategies
may reduce anxiety:

Colors   Pastel or light colors may be more soothing than
              dark or bright colors.
Sounds   Pleasant sounds, such as soft music or nature
              sounds, may be calming.
Textures   Pillow, blankets, or other objects in soft textures
              (velvet, chenille, corduroy, etc.) may be held or
              stroked to relieve stress.
Aromas   Some scents (vanilla, orange, lavender, and
              others) have calming properties. The use of
              scented bath products or room sprays is safer
              than burning scented candles or bowls of pot-
              pourri, which may appear edible.

CREATING A SAFE ENVIRONMENT

Safety is an essential requirement of all living environments. The prevention of injury is a goal of great importance to caregivers. For individuals
with dementia, safety risks can be due to cognitive changes in memory
and judgment as well as physical changes in balance and mobility.

Ensuring safety involves a multifaceted approach that reviews
potential hazards in each room. Categories of hazards will be
reviewed, and a room-by-room guide follows.

Breakable objects	*—Remove glass, ceramic figurines, and other items that could have sharp pieces when broken, or place out of reach.*
Knives	*—Remove knives from accessible locations (countertop knife blocks).* *Consider a locked drawer for storage.*
Matches/Lighters	*—Keep matches and lighters in a locked area.* *Supervise the individual while smoking.*
Guns	*—It is not sufficient to just unload the gun or use a trigger lock.* *—Keep guns and ammunition in separate locked areas.*
Medications/ Vitamins	*—In the early stages of illness, monitor medication usage for accuracy.* *—Try a medication organizer.* *—In later stages, keep medication in a locked area to prevent accidental overdose.*
Household poisons	*—Keep cleaning products and other toxic substances (such as pesticides) in a secure location to prevent accidental consumption.*
Liquor	*—For those who consume alcoholic beverages, monitor rate and amount of consumption to prevent intoxication, which can lead to falls and injury.*
Poisonous plants	*—Some plants and flowers are toxic if ingested. Remove these plants from the environment. Consult your local poison control center for a list of poisonous plants in your area.*
Appliances	*—Unplug irons, hair dryers, and other appliances when not in use.* *—In later stages, supervise use of appliances to prevent injury.*
Power tools	*—In early stages, make sure protective equipment (safety goggles, gloves) are used, and monitor tools use.* *—In later stages, access to tools may need to be restricted.*
Telephones	*—Some individuals with dementia become victims of telemarketing scams. Some caregivers*

	turn down the ringer volume on the telephone before leaving the house, so the individual with dementia does not hear incoming calls.
Summoning help	*—Some individuals are unable to dial 911 for assistance.*
	Consider a pendant-style alarm system, if the individual is capable of learning how to activate such an alarm, and a Safe Return identification bracelet (available through the Alzheimer's Association).
Bathroom doors	*—Some individuals accidentally lock themselves in the bathroom, and can't unlock the door. Consider removing the bathroom door lock, or changing to a lock that can be opened from the outside with a key.*
	—If the bathroom door swings into the bathroom, and the individual falls, she could block access into the bathroom for a caregiver coming to assist her. Consider changing the swing of the door out to the hallway or room instead of into the bathroom.

FALLING HAZARDS

Older adults are at higher risks for falls than the general population due to many changes associated with the aging process. Diminished vision, slowed balance reactions, muscular weakness, and low blood pressure can be contributing factors to falls. For individuals with FTD, decreased judgment and safety awareness, impulsivity, and poor motor planning are also fall risk factors.

The following environmental (extrinsic) factors may lead to falls:

- Lighting that is too dark, too dim, has a glare, or promotes shadows
- Walking surfaces that are uneven, wet/slippery, have busy patterns, have worn carpets or area rugs that are not secured in place, or are waxed floors

- Stairs with edges that are not defined, have uneven riser height, lack of handrails, or wobbly handrails
- Furniture that is too low, too soft, unstable (easily tips or moves), or in the walking path
- Clothing that is too long or too loose
- Footwear that is too loose, has slippery soles, or is unfastened/untied
- Objects on the floor, such as magazine racks, trash cans, small ottomans, or low coffee tables

The solutions to most of the above environmental hazards are simple, and many are no or low-cost interventions. Please see the room-by-room section of this chapter for further safety ideas.

The following physical (intrinsic) factors can increase the risk of falls:

- Medications: sedatives, sleeping aids, some blood pressure reducers
- Being tired/Having insomnia: individuals are more likely to fall when fatigued
- Vision disorders: limited vision can lead to falls
- Ataxia/Balance disorders/Unsteady gait
- Depression
- Poor initiation
- Foot problems
- Fear of falling
- Use of alcohol
- Sedentary lifestyle/Inactivity

Your medical care team (neurologist, physiatrist, ophthalmologist, physical therapist, occupational therapist, etc.) can assist with strategies to minimize the impact of these fall risk factors.

CREATING ENVIRONMENTS THAT MAXIMIZE FUNCTIONAL SKILLS

Environments can support independence when they are designed to provide cues to compensate for declining cognitive skills. This is an ongoing process that changes with the course of the disease. Cues that work in the early stages may be confusing in the later stages. There are several strategies to accomplish this goal; several are listed below.

In the early stages of the disease, labeling drawers with a picture or description of the contents can assist an individual in finding objects used in everyday activities. For example, labeling the utensil drawer in the kitchen with a picture of a fork, or the word "forks" in large letters may enable the individual to find the forks when preparing to set the table.

Leaving commonly used items within sight may help in the early stages of the disease. In the bathroom, leaving the toothpaste and toothbrush on the counter may cue the individual to brush his teeth; leaving a hairbrush may prompt the individual to brush his hair. In the middle stages, having too many items in view may be distracting, and the individual may not be able to determine which items are used for a certain task. He may try to brush his hair with the toothbrush if all the above items are still in view. At that stage, only one item should be left in sight at a time.

The use of grab bars in the bathroom can promote continued ability to transfer to the toilet or bathtub. Grab bars should always be of a contrasting color to the wall on which they are placed for maximum effectiveness.

Use color to highlight or minimize attention to areas of the house. Use a solid contrasting color on the wall behind the toilet to direct attention in the bathroom. Paint a door that you do not want opened in the same color as the rest of the wall, so it appears to blend into the wall.

TECHNOLOGY AND HOME ENVIRONMENTS

Advances in technology can provide assistance in promoting safety and functional skills. Motion detectors can automatically turn on lights as one approaches the bathroom or staircase, or sound an alarm when an individual attempts to leave the house.

These devices are widely available in electronics stores, and the price of these devices is surprisingly affordable.

HOUSEHOLD CHECKLIST

Using the following checklist is a good way to start a home assessment. Some modifications to the home and the related equipment are reimbursable by health insurance plans, including Medicare. The following list has been noted by a double asterisk (**) where the modification or equipment is reimbursable by some health insurance plans. A single asterisk (*) notes items that are non-reimbursable by most health insurance plans. There are other options for funding home modifications besides health insurance. Some have age and income qualifications (CDA Block Grants administered by local Agencies on Aging, Christmas in April, Volunteers in Medical Engineering, benevolent organizations, etc.), others are available only in certain areas (university projects, demonstration grants, etc.). Another option for those that own their own homes is a home equity loan or reverse mortgage.

Bathroom

Are throw rugs secured with double-sided tape?
Is there a nonskid mat, strips, or finish on the tub/shower floor?*
Is there a shower chair?*
Is there a handheld shower?*
Are there grab bars to provide support during transfers and while bathing?*
Are the grab bars in the proper location for the individual?*
Are the grab bars in a contrasting color to the wall?*
Are there grab bars near the toilet?*
Is a raised toilet seat needed?**
Is there sufficient lighting in the bathroom?
Is there a ground fault interrupted (GFI) outlet to avoid electrical shocks while using an electric shaver, hair dryer, or other appliances in the bathroom?*
Is there a phone to summon help if needed?

Bedroom

Is the bed the proper height for the individual?
Is a hospital-style bed needed?**
Is the room cluttered with furniture and accessories?
Is there a place to sit while dressing, other than the bed?

Is there too much clothing in the drawers and closet?
Is there a commode for safer toileting, especially during night time?**
Are there night lights?*

Kitchen

Are there childproof locks on all areas containing hazards?*
Is a range cut-off switch needed to prevent use of the stove or oven?*
Is a refrigerator lock needed?

Stairs

Are there handrails on each side of the steps?*
Are the steps even?
If there is carpeting on the steps, is it firmly attached?
Are there nonskid, contrasting edges on the steps?*
Is the lighting sufficient at the top and bottom of the staircase?
Are there unsecured throw rugs at the top or bottom of the staircase?

Living Room

If carpeted, is the carpeting low pile or are there plastic runners over the
    carpeting to create level paths?*
Is there a clear path to maneuver around furniture?*
Is there a chair with a firm seat and sturdy arms in which to sit?
Is there a lift chair or cushion for easier sitting to standing?** (requires
    a letter of medical necessity)
Is there a glare control at the windows?*

Throughout the Home

Is the home able to accommodate an individual in a wheelchair?
Is one-floor living a possibility? Is there a full bathroom and room for a
    bedroom on the first floor?
Can stair glides be rented or purchased for safer negotiation of stairs and
    to continue access to two floors?*
Is a rented or purchased wheelchair needed for more energy-efficient,
    longer distance mobility?** (Most insurance plans will reimburse
    one wheelchair every five years unless there is medical justification.)
Would a ceiling-based track lift system* or Hoyer lift** system facilitate
    transfers?
Are there one-touch on/off lamps and glow-in-the-dark light switches?*

INTERNET RESOURCES

Abledata—database of assistive devices and manufacturer/distributor information. www.abledata.com.

Adaptive Environments Center—home modification resources. www.adaptenv.org.

Ageless Design—great information on dementia-specific home modifications. www.agelessdesign.com.

American Association for Retired Persons (AARP)—general information about home modifications. www.aarp.org

American Occupational Therapy Association—information on home modification and how to contact an occupational therapist. www.aota.org.

LifeEase—home evaluation information. www.lifease.com.

National Resource Center on Supportive Housing and Home Modifications, University of Southern California, Andrus Gerontology Center—home modification information. www.homemods.org.

NOTES

1. E. C. Brawley, "Environment—A Silent Partner in Caregiving," in *Behaviors in Dementia: Best Practices for Successful Management*, ed. M. Kaplan and S. B. Hoffman (Baltimore, Md.: Health Promotions Press, 1998).

2. R. V. Olsen, E. Ehrenkratz, and B. Hutchings, *Homes That Help* (Newark, N.J.: NJIT Press, 1993).

BIBLIOGRAPHY

Brawley, E. C. *Designing for Alzheimer's Disease: Strategies for Creating Better Care Environments.* New York: John Wiley and Sons, 1997.

Calkins, M. P. *Creating Successful Dementia Care Settings.* Baltimore: Health Professions Press, 2001.

Changing Needs, Changing Homes: A Guide to Resources. Bethesda, Md.: American Occupational Therapy Foundation and American Occupational Therapy Association, 1996.

Pynoos, J., J. Sanford, and T. Rosenfelt. "A team approach for home modification." *OT Practice* 7, no. 7 (2002): 15–19.

Ruga, W. "Designing for the Senses." In *Healthcare Design*, edited by S. Marberry. New York: John Wiley and Sons, 1997.

Sanford, L. "The importance of lighting for the elderly." *Aging and Vision* 11, no. 1 (1999) (Available online at www.lighthouse.org.).

Warner, M. L. *The Complete Guide to Alzheimer's-Proofing Your Home.* West Lafayette, Ind.: Purdue University Press, 2000.

Wylde, M., A. Baron-Robbins, and S. Clark. *Building for a Lifetime.* Newton, Conn.: Tauton, 1994.

CHAPTER 15

Altered Relationships:
Adapting to Emotions and Behavior

KATHERINE P. RANKIN

INTRODUCTION

As you have probably realized from the previous chapters in this volume, one of the most important differences between the frontotemporal dementia syndromes and Alzheimer's disease is that the frontal dementias primarily affect behavior, often early and severely. It is this factor, perhaps more than any other, that makes caring for a frontal dementia sufferer so much more of a challenge. To make things even more complicated, the experiences among FTD caregivers differ considerably, because the areas of the brain that are damaged in the frontal dementias vary substantially from patient to patient. One caregiver may be at the end of his rope because he finds himself battling the patient over her excessively rigid, compulsive eating behavior. Another may find that though her loved one is easy-going and complacent, she dreads taking him into public places due to his tendency to make loud, socially inappropriate comments to strangers and friends. As the disease progresses, particular behavioral changes may appear and then disappear later in a manner that researchers are only beginning to understand, much less be able to predict. However, as this family of diseases becomes more widely recognized by the public and the scientific community alike, new resources are becoming available to alleviate some of the burden and isolation experienced by FTD caregivers in the past.

205

This chapter will describe some of the social and emotional changes particular to dementia patients whose disease affects the frontal and/or temporal lobes of the brain, and make some suggestions about how to cope with or manage these changes. These symptoms are commonly found in frontotemporal dementia patients but will also sometimes occur in other diseases such as corticobasal degeneration and progressive supranuclear palsy. There already exists literature directed toward dementia caregiving that can provide very helpful guidance in the major principles of behavior management. However, there are a few issues that are worth briefly repeating here. During the course of their loved one's dementia, caregivers will experience a series of changes in the patient's manner and behavior over time. The first important step for the caregiver is to learn to notice each change, no matter how gradually it has appeared. This is not only necessary to give the patient's healthcare providers accurate information to aid in treatment decisions, but it is an important issue for maintaining a healthy caregiving relationship. For each change, caregivers must first ask, "How is this behavior affecting quality of life for me, the patient, and others around us?" Second, they must ask, "Is the best course of action to (1) adjust to this new behavior, (2) try to change it, or (3) both?" Caregivers must recognize that not every challenging new behavior really needs to be changed, nor will it even be possible given the nature of the patient's disease. Conversely, however, caregivers must also be honest about the negative impact a behavior may be having upon themselves or others, and should not choose to overburden themselves unnecessarily by neglecting opportunities to either modify the patient's challenging behavior or obtain additional assistance coping with it. Above all, caregiving for frontal dementia patients requires flexibility and an awareness that each new problem may need to be handled using a different approach than the problem before.

For instance, a patient may develop an affinity for a particular shirt, and will insist on wearing that shirt and no other. After a few weeks of escalating conflict over her attempts to dress the patient differently, one caregiver may decide that, other than the mild embarrassment it causes her in social settings, this behavior is having no negative effects on the patient or others. This caregiver chooses to wash the shirt regularly and ceases her attempts to make the patient wear other shirts, thus resolving the problem by choosing to adjust to the behavior rather than change it. For a different caregiver, however, the added effort of laundering the favorite shirt three to four times per week would be an unreasonable drain on her limited time and energy, and she may opt for a compromise. She agrees to allow the patient to wear the same color and style of shirt daily, adapting to his wishes despite her embarrassment, but will buy five identical versions of the shirt for the patient to wear. If the patient is bothered by the fact that these are in fact different shirts, it still may require some effort and creativity on the part of the caregiver to convince him to wear them. However, working to slightly modify the patient's behavior will significantly decrease her workload and help protect her quality of life.

The second main caregiving principle that should be reiterated here is that it is crucial for caregivers to monitor themselves and know when to get help. Numerous studies suggest that it is a dementia patient's behavioral disturbance, not her cognitive decline (e.g., poor memory or mental disorganization), that is the most significant predictor of social and emotional distress for the caregiver.[1] Clearly, this issue is particularly salient in the case of frontal dementia caregivers, as the social and behavioral manifestations of the disease are often the primary symptoms and challenge the caregiver on a daily basis. The suggestions entailed in this chapter are only an initial resource for handling the strain of caring for a frontal dementia patient. Chapters 18 through 22 of this volume are dedicated to elucidating the resources available to provide support for caregivers when the patient's emotional and social behaviors become too much to handle alone.

INSIGHT AND AWARENESS

Loss of self-awareness is one of the hallmarks of FTD, and it is often one of the most difficult aspects of the disease for caregivers. Patients can have problems recognizing that they are ill, or may appear to be unable to correctly monitor their own behavior or their impact on others. In fact, when frontal dementia patients are asked to describe their current personality and behaviors, many will state that there is "nothing wrong with them" and will describe themselves as they once were, even misreporting factual information about themselves. Though the family members report, for instance, that this once genial and extroverted woman has become persistently harsh, critical, and uninterested in social engagements, the patient's self-description will match the family's report of her extroverted and pleasant personality before the onset of the disease. She may even say that she likes to go to parties regularly when she has not been willing to attend such an event for years. It is important to realize that this is not a case of psychological denial, as if the patient refuses to admit changes that could be perceived as shortcomings. This is, in fact, a brain-based disorder that prevents patients from accurately perceiving and interpreting new information about their behavior that would challenge their longstanding self-image.

This problem can result from damage to various structures in the right hemisphere of the brain, which is believed to be the location of complex circuits that process and update information about one's physical and emotional state, personal history, and interpersonal relationships. It has long been demonstrated that patients who have strokes damaging the right parietal lobe can lose awareness of their own disease or dysfunction. It can be to the point where a paralyzed patient will insist that he has never been immobilized, or a blind patient will state that she can see and will create elaborate, inaccurate descriptions of her surroundings. This lack of awareness of one's disease, or "anosognosia," is often seen in Alzheimer's patients, probably because the parietal lobe typically becomes damaged as a part of this disease. However, patients with damage to the frontal or temporal lobes of the brain also can evidence anosognosia, even without parietal damage, and researchers are still searching for the specific neuroanatomic origins of this loss of insight. Recent studies of a structure in the upper middle of the frontal lobe, the anterior cingulate, suggest that it is involved in helping an individual to actively address their internal information stores.[2] The anterior cingulate is severely damaged in the frontal variant of FTD, and sustains some damage in the temporal variant.[3] Interestingly, recent studies suggest that the cingulate is relatively spared in the progressive aphasia (left frontal) subtype of FTD,[4] the only subtype in which patients typically retain full awareness of their disease and maintain normal social behavior until late in the disease process.

Caregivers learning to cope with a frontal dementia patient's lack of insight may find that their frustration is partly alleviated when they accept that it will be difficult, if not impossible, for the patient to recognize the truth about himself and his behavior. This is merely a part of the dementia, just as failure to lay down new memories is a part of Alzheimer's disease. Maintaining patience and compassion is key. A caregiver's attempts to hold up a mirror to the patient will often result in escalating a fruitless power struggle. And yet, caregivers should also recognize that the patient's lack of self-awareness may actually be a blessing in disguise. This lack of insight actually presents much more of a burden for the caregiver than for the patient, who is oblivious to what would probably be devastating information about their progressive loss of abilities and the dramatic change from their previously held standards of behavior.

The practical issue arising from lack of insight that perhaps carries the greatest potential for harm occurs when the patient refuses to participate in evaluation and treatment due to their failure to recognize their illness. At our dementia specialty clinic, I have witnessed instances where the family members were eventually forced to deceive the patient about the true purpose of the visit to convince the patient to cooperate with necessary medical treatment. The ethical issues involved in the treatment of dementia patients are often thorny; however, when it comes to the point where deception and coercion seem necessary, the patient's lack of insight may be interfering with her capacity to make decisions in her best interest. To resolve this issue, the primary caregiver may choose to seek legal guardianship of the patient to be allowed to make medical decisions for her. With an FTD patient who manifests this lack of insight early in the disease, before other functional impairments arise, it may require testimony from a specialist in frontotemporal dementia to convince the legal authorities that the patient should have a conservator. (See chapter 21 for more information.) In all such cases, it is important to thoroughly discuss the issue with the treatment team to determine a course of action that maximizes the dignity and independence of the patient while maintaining appropriate standards for his care.

LOSS OF EMPATHY

Another change that can come as a shock, particularly to family and friends, is that some FTD patients lose their ability to sense what others are feeling, and may become extraordinarily self-centered as a part of their disease. One caregiver described an incident in which he had cut off part of his toe with a lawnmower. He was appalled when his wife casually walked over to the neighbor's house to return the borrowed mower before getting into the car to drive to the hospital. While in the car, she showed no distress over his injury and even told him he was "making too much noise." In another incident, a caregiver who had been very close to his mother before her disease tried to convey to her some very difficult times he'd been having at work. His mother was so preoccupied with turning the topic back to the mundane events of her day that even when the son began to cry describing an incident he had experienced, his mother merely looked bewildered for a moment, then returned to chatting away about her garden. Both of these patients were early in their disease, and neither had yet been diagnosed with frontotemporal dementia, though they were both later found to have the temporal variant of FTD.

This decreased emotional responsiveness is a direct result of change to certain structures in the brain. The amygdala, a structure found inside of the temporal lobes, is responsible for producing emotions such as fear and anger, and helps us to recognize emotion in others' faces and voices. This structure is damaged early and severely in some types of FTD, even to the point where a structural MRI scan shows only a large hole in the brain where that structure should be. Again, researchers are only beginning to understand how amygdala loss contributes to emotional blunting and loss of empathy in FTD patients, but it appears that damage to the right side of the brain is more likely to cause difficulty with emotional receptivity and expression.[5] Recent evidence suggests that the right temporal lobe is also involved with higher-level interpretation of emotional signals originating from the amygdala.[6] Thus, damage to parts of the right temporal lobe can interfere with the patient's capacity to realize that certain facial expressions, body postures, gestures, and voice inflections carry emotional significance, making them unable to recognize others' emotions or correctly interpret social signals.

Research also suggests that right temporal damage may disrupt the ability to recognize when a situation or memory is supposed to have personal emotional relevance, causing some patients to lose their sense of attachment to loved ones.[7] If this problem is compounded by a lack of insight, the patient will not only fail to correctly identify the emotional state of the other, but they will not even realize that they are missing something. This is also one of the reasons some FTD patients make inappropriate or judgmental comments to friends or strangers, or insist on conversation topics that do not interest their listeners. Initial reports suggest that patients with temporal lobe damage are more likely to be perceived as unempathic, aloof, and even cold-hearted by their caregivers than patients whose damage is predominantly in the frontal lobes.[8] However, the emotion system is also disrupted in frontal patients,[9] and both types become extremely introverted socially. In both temporal and frontal variants of FTD there is extensive damage to the lower middle part of the frontal lobes, called the orbitofrontal cortex, another part of the brain that is highly connected with the amygdala and which helps to mediate socially appropriate behavior. Also, though frontal patients appear to be better at recognizing emotions than temporal patients, they also tend to be much more apathetic and are less likely to give any response in a social interaction.

Humans are by nature social, relational beings, and we tend to gauge who people are by how they interact with us. Thus, the emotional blunting and loss of emotional attachment that occurs in many FTD patients can make caregivers feel like they are living with a stranger. Again, coping with this change begins with a clear recognition that this is not willful coldness or spitefulness on the part of the patient, but is a loss of emotional functioning directly caused by damage to the brain. However, it is natural to feel that such patients are more prickly and difficult to like, and the emotional one-sidedness of the relationship puts additional strain on FTD caregivers on a day-to-day basis. Like the loss of insight described previously, loss of empathic warmth cannot be changed through behavioral interventions, and caregivers must shoulder the burden of adapting to the patient's change in personality. One of the most important things caregivers can do in this situation is to make an honest assessment of the way this change affects them emotionally, and to give themselves the opportunity to mourn this loss. A readjustment of the caregiver's support system is often necessary, recruiting other family members, friends, community, and counselors to provide the nurture and emotional attentiveness that the patient can no longer supply. Studies show that when family members can learn to view the caregiving relationship with greater distance, taking on a perspective similar to that which is held by nonrelative caregivers, they become happier, better adjusted, and more effective caregivers.[10] Though many FTD patients show decreased empathy, only a small proportion of them become entirely incapable of emotional expression or receptivity, thus most caregivers will still occasionally experience some modified emotional responsiveness from the patient. When a caregiver ceases to expect direct emotional support from the patient and his emotional needs are adequately met elsewhere, they are more likely to appreciate and even enjoy the patient again, making the caregiving relationship less stressful.

APATHY

Another change that may be seen in patients with dementias affecting the frontal lobes of the brain is loss of interest in the activities and people that they used to enjoy. In frontotemporal dementia patients, this apathy is usually distinct from depression, though the two are easily confused by family members and clinicians. Both apathy and depression may cause a decrease in activity, loss of interest and enjoyment, and a general lack of responsiveness. However, typical depression is characterized by somatic symptoms such as loss of appetite, weight loss, and insomnia, as well as negative cognitive preoccupations with worthlessness, hopelessness, sadness, and helplessness. Rather than becoming more preoccupied with negative emotions and thoughts, however, FTD patients with apathy actually cease to be troubled by the things that used to bother them. They begin to generate fewer thoughts and emotions, and initiate fewer words and actions. Families of FTD patients will sometimes report that their first indication that something was wrong was that the patient *stopped* worrying and became uncharacteristically complacent and passive. A patient who has been hardworking and conscientious her whole life may suddenly stop bothering to meet deadlines or may quit her job altogether without cause or explanation.

Later in the disease, this apathy may become so pervasive that she only speaks when spoken to and moves only when led around, showing very little interest in the events and conversations going on around her, even when she herself is the topic of discussion.

The brain structure that most likely is responsible for apathy is the anterior cingulate, a band of tissue in the middle of the frontal cortex. Patients with strokes limited to this brain area sometimes develop what is called "akinetic mutism," a severe form of apathy where the patient stops moving and speaking altogether despite intact brain systems for language and movement. Studies have directly linked apathy with anterior cingulate damage in frontotemporal dementia patients.[11] Though about half of temporal variant patients show increased apathy (an equivalent increase is seen in patients with Alzheimer's disease), 95 percent of patients with the frontal variant of FTD show increased apathy.[12] Research suggests that the anterior cingulate is involved with extroversion[13] and with actively addressing information from internal sources.[14] Functional imaging studies show that the lower portions of the anterior cingulate can be hyperactive in patients with depression or anxiety,[15] perhaps in conjunction with their negative, ruminative thought patterns. The fact that this structure is significantly atrophied in frontal variant FTD suggests that patients' apathy may result from an incapacity to derive motivation from internal cues.

Apathy can be both a curse and a blessing for caregivers. On the one hand, patients cease to be supportive and helpful in the household, often requiring prompting to perform basic self-care tasks, much less do work around the home. They can become dependent and passive, putting more of a burden on caregivers to step into the role of provider, organizer, and director in the relationship. This can be a particularly difficult transition when the patient once had the dominant role in the relationship, such as in the case of a breadwinner or parent. At first caregivers may be very reluctant to perform the coaching and prompting that is often necessary with apathetic patients, and may find that they need to develop previously unexplored skills, such as attending to financial concerns or housework. On the other hand, apathy tends to make patients more compliant and cooperative with care and treatment, and they are less likely to engage in power struggles with caregivers. Depending upon the degree of apathy, some patients actually become much more easygoing, pleasant, and even more friendly than they were before the onset of their disease. Patients are spared the pain of caring about their condition, and remain comparatively untroubled despite significant loss of function and freedom. When asked how they feel, apathetic patients will typically respond genuinely that they feel "just fine" and that their symptoms are not bothering them.

Again, the origin of apathy in frontotemporal dementia patients is entirely neurologic and not psychological, and thus is not subject to rehabilitation; however, there are some behavioral interventions that may make it easier for caregivers to manage patients. Even in patients for whom the apathy is pervasive, they typically have some preserved likes and dislikes that can be utilized as concrete motivators or rewards. The typical scenario with a very apathetic patient is that the caregiver wishes for the patient to do something, for example, get dressed or bathe, and the patient would really rather not. In such a case, if the caregiver has noted that the patient likes a particular food or television show, she can promise this as a reward for performing the task. Though the patient's cognitive deficits may keep him from focusing on the reward long enough to complete the task, the caregiver may wish to frequently remind the patient of the imminent reward to prime his deficient motivational system. At other times, however, the caregiver must take a good look at her reasons for wanting the patient to perform a particular task, and she may need to adjust her expectations. For example, she may decide that since the patient is no longer attending regular social events or going to work daily, more infrequent bathing may be adequate and appropriate.

RIGID, BIZARRE, AND SOCIALLY INAPPROPRIATE BEHAVIOR

Perhaps the most infamous aspect of the frontal dementia syndromes is their tendency to produce odd behavior in some patients. Some patients will develop compulsive behaviors such as playing computer solitaire for hours every day, insisting on eating only very specific foods, or buying a favorite object every time they find one at the store (e.g., pens, stepladders, cans of soup). This compulsivity is often accompanied by mental rigidity, where patients have certain ideas about how things must be done and are highly resistant to alternatives. They may also become obsessed with a particular place, event, or theme, and will persistently bring the conversation back around to this topic even when listeners have no interest in it or even remind the patient that they have heard the story many times before. Some patients will develop odd or repetitive movements, such as fidgeting, pacing, walking oddly for no discernable medical reason, putting inedible objects in their mouth, or grimacing. Other patients will show a disregard for social norms, touching themselves or others inappropriately, making inappropriate or rude comments, stealing, or wearing bizarre clothing combinations.

Neuroanatomically, these behaviors are commonly believed to be linked to the right hemisphere of the brain, particularly the frontal and temporal lobes, but beyond that their mechanisms are not very well understood. Research suggests that patients with damage to the right orbitofrontal area of the frontal lobe may retain the capacity to accurately describe and explain social norms, but can no longer behave appropriately despite this knowledge. Impulse control is also mediated by various circuits in the frontal lobes, including the orbitofrontal cortex and the anterior cingulate, and is frequently deficient in FTD. These more bizarre behaviors can sometimes be controlled by using pharmacological treatment to increase an important neurotransmitter that is commonly diminished in frontotemporal dementia. That neurotransmitter is serotonin. In particular, compulsive behavior, irritability, impulsivity, and the tendency to consume excessive amounts of sweets and other carbohydrates often respond to treatment with psychotropic medications.[16]

This category of behavior can cause more frustration, annoyance, and embarrassment for caregivers than any other. As with many other aspects of the disease, caregivers must simply learn to live with some of these behaviors. And, they must make sure to monitor their own level of irritation and find a friend or family member who is willing to provide respite care when the patient's behavior becomes too much to take. However, there are some behavioral interventions that can either modify or limit the effects of the patient's behavior:

- Some caregivers find that it is helpful to carry a set of preprinted, business-card-sized notes for use in situations where the patient behaves oddly or inappropriately in public. Such a card could read, "My wife has an Alzheimer's-like disease that affects her behavior. Thank you for your patience," and could be handed unobtrusively to the food server who receives an undeserved rambling lecture from the patient, or the stranger whose attire is commented upon a little too loudly.

- Patients who steal items typically do so impulsively rather than because they actually need the item in question. If the caregiver is familiar with the patient's interests and habits, it will become easier to recognize environments that may contain objects the patient might be tempted to steal (certain types of stores, friends' homes, passing by street vendors with open display cases). Patients may require extra supervision in such environments. It may be helpful to recruit the help of a second caregiver to monitor the patient if the primary caregiver will be otherwise occupied. Sometimes, physically placing oneself between the patient and the display rack is enough of a deterrent. Also, discreetly checking the patient for stolen items before or immediately after leaving the problem environment may sometimes be necessary to minimize unwanted consequences.

- Though rigid, compulsive behavior is by nature resistant to change, compromises can sometimes be reached by bargaining with patients. (Anecdotally, I have heard some caregivers of patients with empathy deficits indicate that their loved ones have begun to drive very hard, somewhat unfair bargains as a result of their disease, so proceed with caution!) Again, this requires having a clear understanding of the patient's interests and preoccupations. The goal is to convince the patient to give up one desire (e.g., buying a fifth set of socket wrenches) to be rewarded with another (e.g., sitting for a half hour in the food court of the mall while the patient plays solitaire on a handheld computer game). It is always a good idea to plan ahead to minimize the need to push or rush the patient. Expect even simple activities to require more time than they once did. For instance, some caregivers choose to schedule an extra hour in the morning on the day of an appointment so they can negotiate with any of the patient's unanticipated demands or rituals without being late.

NOTES

1. A. Braekhus et al., "Social and depressive stress suffered by spouses of patients with mild dementia," *Scandinavian Journal of Primary Health Care* 16, no. 4 (1998): 242–46; M. Bedard et al., "Associations between dysfunctional behaviors, gender, and burden in spousal caregivers of cognitively impaired older adults," *International Psychogeriatrics* 9, no. 3 (1997): 277–90; L. D. Clyburn et al., "Predicting caregiver burden in Alzheimer's disease," *Journal of Gerontology* 55B, no. 1 (2000): S2–S13; C. Donaldson, N. Tarrier, and A. Burns, "Determinants of career stress in Alzheimer's disease," *International Journal of Geriatric Psychiatry* 13 (1998): 248–56.

2. D. Ebert and K. P. Ebmeier, "The role of the cingulate gyrus in depression: From functional anatomy to neurochemistry," *Biological Psychiatry* 39 (1996): 1044–50.

3. H. J. Rosen et al., "Patterns of brain atrophy in frontotemporal dementia and semantic dementia," *Neurology* 58, no. 2 (2002): 198–208.

4. M. L. Gorno-Tempini, personal communication.

5. H. J. Rosen et al., "Emotion comprehension in the temporal variant of frontotemporal dementia," *Brain* 125 (2002): 2286–95; R. J. Perry et al., "Hemispheric dominance for emotions, empathy, and social behaviour: Evidence from right and left handers with frontotemporal dementia," *Neurocase* 7, no. 2 (2001): 145–60.

6. T. Allison, A. Puce, and G. McCarthy, "Social perception from visual cues: Role of the STS region," *Trends in Cognitive Sciences* 4, no. 7 (2000): 267–78; R. Adolphs, "Social cognition and the human brain," *Trends in Cognitive Sciences* 3, no. 12 (1999): 469–79.

7. D. Van Lancker, "Personal relevence and the human right hemisphere," *Brain and Cognition* 17 (1991): 64–92.

8. K. P. Rankin et al., "Double dissociation of social functioning in frontotemporal dementia," *Neurology* 60, no. 2 (2003): 266–71.

9. P. Mychack, J. Kramer, and B. Miller, "Lateralization of facial affect in frontotemporal dementia," *Archives of Clinical Neuropsychology* 15, no. 8 (2000): 742–43.

10. K. W. Hepburn et al., "Dementia family caregiver training: Affecting beliefs about caregiving and caregiver outcomes," *Journal of the American Geriatric Society* 49 (2001): 450–57.

11. W. Liu et al., "Behavioral disorders in the frontal and temporal variants of frontotemporal lobar degeneration," n.d.

12. K. P. Rankin, "Anatomy of depression: Teaching from studies of frontotemporal disorders," paper presented at the XXIII Congress of the Collegium Internationale Neuropsychopharmacologicum, Montreal, Canada, 2002.

13. K. P. Ebmeier et al., "Personality associations with the uptake of the cerebral blood flow marker 99mTc-Exametazime estimated wth single photon emission tomography," *Personality and Individual Differences* 17 (1994): 587–95.

14. I. J. Deary et al., "PASAT performance and the pattern of uptake of 99mTc-Exametazime in the brain estimated with single photon emission tomography," *Biological Psychology* 38 (1994): 1–18.

15. D. Ebert et al., "Single photon emission computerized tomography assessment of cerebral dopamine D2 receptor blockade in depression before and after sleep deprivation: Preliminary results," *Biological Psychiatry* 35 (1994): 880–85.

16. R. J. Perry and B. L. Miller "Behavior and treatment in frontotemporal dementia," *Neurology* 56 (11 Suppl 4) (2001): S46–S51.

CHAPTER 16

A Balance of Health:
Maintaining General Medical Care Practices

BRUCE L. MILLER AND ROSALIE GEARHART

What will he be like after surgery?
Is cancer screening important at this point?
If the test is positive, what will happen next?
What are the alternatives?

The goal of this chapter is to outline some guiding principles to support you through the ongoing decision-making process regarding health issues as a caregiver for a person with FTD. Because FTD is still a relatively understudied disorder, there are few research studies or tested theories that are available to guide you. We all learn as we go along this difficult journey, and much of what is shared in this chapter comes from the experiences, stories, and writings of patients and families who have waged a fight against this devastating illness. They have championed this cause to help others avoid the traumatic experiences that they have gone through with FTD. Due to their courage, we are fast approaching the day when we will no longer receive calls from caregivers reporting "they don't know much about FTD around here."

This chapter is based on the overarching goal of helping caregivers make effective decisions for their loved one. Rarely in the caregiving world do we take the time to reflect on how we got here and how we worked through so many difficult decisions. How do we know what is the right thing to do? Simply stated, there is no single right answer. Rather, we always need to take a step backward to think about how to tailor care based upon the individual's values and preferences, ethnicity, cultural background, and spiritual practices. The lifetime of conversations and joint experiences, and the shared family values will give you special insights that no physician, nurse, social worker, or psychologist will have. Your own instincts will serve you well!

Of course, caregiving for FTD is a job that no one ever expected, so usually there has been no training for this role, and no prior planning. Initially, the addition of caregiver duties to existing family responsibilities can be overwhelming. It is hard enough to make up our own minds about our personal health choices, but what do we do when someone else's mind is changing so that we need to make decisions for them as well? And what do we do when that person is no longer able to discuss their preferences and participate effectively in healthcare decisions?

The guidelines and principles outlined in this chapter can help you to structure an organized and focused approach to anticipated and unanticipated healthcare decisions. It is important for patients, families, and clinicians to make decisions together about treatment plans and treatment goals. Caring for an impaired individual requires a team that will divide the work that is required to accomplish the plan. There will be a stage when joint decisions with the patient are no longer possible. Ongoing assessment and input from the clinicians involved will help to determine when this occurs and you need not feel like you must handle any decision alone. You should choose your physician and other advisors carefully so that you are comfortable with their advice. (See chapter 4 for more information.) Finally, it is important to have realistic expectations for the ill person as the disease progresses.

PATIENTS' RIGHTS

All healthcare organizations adopt some version of patients' rights for staff to follow in the delivery of care to patients. Patients' rights were first developed in response to the need to ensure consistent and fair care to all. In response to the special needs of dementia patients and their families, caregivers have developed an Alzheimer's disease Bill of Rights.

- to have appropriate, ongoing medical care
- to be productive in work and play as long as possible
- to be treated like an adult, not like a child
- to have expressed feelings taken seriously
- to be free from psychotrophic medications if possible
- to live in a safe, structured, and predictable environment
- to enjoy meaningful activities that fill each day
- to be outdoors on a regular basis
- to have physical contact, including hugging, caressing, and hand-holding
- to be individuals who know our life's story including cultural and religious traditions
- to be cared for by individuals who are well trained in dementia care

You are a key person in assessing the patients' ability to make decisions for themselves along with the professional healthcare providers. This requires an ongoing assessment that can be guided by the following questions. Among the many losses patients with dementia inevitably experience is loss of competency to make decisions for themselves.

- What is the patient's understanding of the illness?
- What is the patient's current level of participation in his care?
- Can the patient show an appreciation of the risks and the benefits involved?
- Can the patient provide rational reasons for the decision?

Patients' rights are available to you to support your advocacy for your loved ones across all settings: clinics, hospitals, assistive living facilities, and long-term care facilities. This all means you are not alone in this process.

ETHICAL PRINCIPLES

The moral principles involved in dementia care have been widely reviewed in the bioethical literature. Many novel terms have been developed specific to the progressive degenerative nature of the diseases. Dementia-specific terms regarding competence and treatments that extend the course but do not cure the disease—such as "the then self" and "negotiated autonomy" are used by ethicists. Ethical principles are utilized to govern care and to lead one's life. Often there are conflicts between one, or more than one, of the bioethical principles of autonomy, confidentiality, truth telling, beneficence, and justice when caring for a demented person. These conflicts come up regularly in day-to-day decisions. For example, it is common to see an FTD patient who wants to continue to drive (autonomy), yet we must also protect his or her personal safety as well as the general public's safety (beneficence). The ethical issues commonly encountered by caregivers in decision making include autonomy, competency, consent, advance directives, truth telling, genetic testing, artificial (tube) feeding, behavior control, research, and end-of-life care.

Most bioethical discussions regarding dementia have focused on professionals. There is little written about the ethical issues from the perspective of family caregivers, yet many of the problems faced by caregivers require the same ethical considerations faced by professionals. Unlike issues for professionals, issues for caregivers arise from a personal context and are often shaped by long-term relationships.

We all use guiding principles and belief systems to live our lives and to relate to others. Our society has established certain rules and norms, many based on our best interests and designed to protect our autonomy. Caring for an adult with dementia often forces us to readdress these principles. As we strive to avoid being overly paternalistic in the delivery of our care, we must also protect the patient from harm or risks that the disease has created secondary to lack of insight, poor judgment, and impaired reasoning.

CAREGIVER ROLES IN HEALTH DECISIONS

Unlike many other adult-onset illnesses, FTD requires that the family play an essential role in the diagnostic process and care on an intimate level. Identifying the roles of all caregivers involved can be helpful in sharing the job. Identify the strengths and, yes, the weaknesses of the caregivers involved. Some family members may have a more sophisticated knowledge of the healthcare delivery systems and they can be identified as the ones to talk with the multiple healthcare providers. Others may have the most patience and empathy and these skills can be used to spend the time providing direct daily care, listening and talking with the patient. It is important to utilize individual expertise and strengths and to constantly reassess whether the family is the best choice as caregiver or if a nonfamily alternative caregiver is indicated. We have found that FTD patients are often made more pliant and trusting by their illness, which, in turn, makes them particularly accepting of new caregivers who are not within the family.

There are no published studies of the reactions, experiences, or burdens involved in caregiving for a loved one with FTD. No doubt, as with Alzheimer's disease, FTD caregiving is an emotional rollercoaster. Adding to this problem is the fact that our society undervalues the role of caregiving. Caregivers may feel proud of their accomplishments, strengthened by their love and commitment to their loved one as well as frustrated, exhausted, and depressed. In everyday life it is difficult to separate the needs and preferences of the patient from the needs and best interests of the caregivers. The effect that caregiving has on the relationship with the patient cannot be overlooked. The value of the family's participation in the healthcare of the patient is indisputable, but is known to place strain on the dynamics of adult relationships. It is important to focus on the strengths of the patients as well as the caregivers. People need acknowledgment of their successes and accomplishments when faced with such challenging situations and stress.

ANTICIPATING HEALTH CARE DECISIONS THROUGH THE COURSE OF THE DISEASE

Early planning for decisions, when possible, is the key to making successful choices and reducing stress. Discussing choices with the patient early in the disease is helpful but can be difficult and sometimes even counterproductive due to the patient's deficits in judgment and insight. Asking help from a professional to guide this discussion can be very constructive and supportive. It is vital to collect information and to ask all the questions you need, but be careful not to let information collection harmfully delay your decisions. It is vital to establish the goals of care based on the current stage of the disease and life expectancy. Each informed decision must weigh the risks and benefits regarding the possible outcomes. The goal is to optimize the level of function and the quality of life for all involved.

Setting the Scene

Whether it is a routine health-related visit or an unexpected visit to the emergency room, some planning and thought will need to be given to ensure the most successful outcomes. Personality and behavioral changes are hallmarks of this disease. As the primary caregiver, you most likely have the best understanding of how your loved one may react during a medical visit. If possible, discuss your needs and concerns ahead of time. Discuss with staff the optimal forms of communication and potential avenues for decision making. Discuss the possible role of medication. Ensure that your loved one feels included in discussions related to her health care. Also, talking to other families of FTD patients may give you additional ideas of what works. Having a durable power of attorney for health care acknowledges the role of the assigned decision maker in the event the person with FTD loses the capacity to make informed decisions. (See chapter 21 for more information.)

Being prepared for the visits to health providers optimizes the use of the face-to-face time with the healthcare provider in an environment where third-party payers (insurance) are shortening the time allotted for visits. Maintain a record of the names of all healthcare providers, their contact information, and the dates of service. It can be very helpful to spend the time to write up the history of the illness so that important details and events are not forgotten. Also keep a list of all medications and note the response to the medications or any side effects and the response when off medications. Maintain health insurance information, policy numbers, and telephone numbers in an organized manner.

Probably one of the most important management tools for caring for a FTD patient is keeping track of any changes in behavior or personality. This behavior log will be extremely helpful to healthcare providers when administering selected treatments and interventions. It is also helpful to caregivers as it assists in identifying patterns or potentially causative factors that may lead to disturbed behaviors. A behavior log can also be very valuable in helping caregivers to realize that it is not their own personal issues at fault. They can quietly sit and review at a calm moment several weeks of notes that clearly confirm their worries and suspicions. FTD is a behaviorally loaded disease, and it can be very challenging to self-reflect and acknowledge your own emotions and reactions to the behaviors of a person with a brain disease that causes drastic changes in expected behaviors and characteristics.

Patients with FTD often have no insight into their condition and, therefore, concerned family members often have a difficult time getting them to seek help. This is where distractions can be of help. Often caregivers will ask the patient to come to the doctor's appointment for another problem that the patient is concerned about. We have had many visits to our memory clinic for knee pain or new glasses. They are important needs to address as well, but certainly not always the primary reason for the visit. Another strategy to get resistant patients into a clinic for help is to refocus their attention on someone else. Ask them to come along for you. Say you need to talk to someone about a problem. Also, since a person with FTD may have a good memory, a promised reward may work as an incentive. For example, a stop at a favorite spot on the trip home may lead to cooperation. Staff at dementia centers can be very helpful. Do not hesitate to call and ask for suggestions or guidance.

Health Maintenance

> *How do I get him to the dentist?*
> *I'm not sure if she can't understand me or can't hear me.*
> *What about alternative treatments?*

A person's values and beliefs, as well as her ability to access care, influence screening for health-related problems. You and your family should develop a close working relationship with your primary care provider to ensure that thoughtful decisions are made that reflect your values and beliefs. In general, the adoption of sound nutritional practices, exercise, and adequate rest promote health and well-being and may help prevent illness and disability. It is also important to remember that, while behavioral changes are a key feature in FTD, sudden changes may indicate an illness such as the flu or urinary infection, or adverse effects of medication, and medical evaluation should be sought. It is critical for all of us to maintain our health at an optimal level. Making sure all sensory systems are functionioning at their best is very important. Routine eye exams, hearing exams, podiatry exams, and dental care can prevent problems and improve quality of life. There are standard health screenings, such as colonoscopy or mammography, that are recommended. Decisions regarding the benefits for these screenings will be based on the stage of the illness and the potential outcomes. For example, a decision to screen for prostate or breast cancer should include a discussion on what will be done if results are positive. Will surgery or treatment be considered or would they not be an option because of the stage of dementia?

Interventions and Treatment

> *What new FTD management issues can be anticipated and when?*
> *What changes are atypical and deserve evaluation for a superimposed problem?*
> *How long will it take before we know the treatment is working?*
> *At what stage of the disease would you consider it inappropriate to continue use of any of the treatment options?*
> *How long will the patient benefit from this invasive procedure?*

There are some general rules to follow when planning treatment and discussing treatment options with healthcare providers. The first is to start with one change at a time. For example, if your loved one is experiencing problems with both mood and cognition and you have decided to use a medication, it is always best to pick the most bothersome problem and to initiate treatment of one problem at a time with one medication at a time. This is the best way to tell whether the medication is having the desired effect. Additional medications may be needed, but when two or more are started at the same time it is difficult to determine which medication is effective or is causing side effects.

Another rule to follow regarding medication usage is to start low and go slow. In this way, the lowest, yet most therapeutic, dose of medication can be used. Also, in selecting pharmacological treatments it is important to consider the simplest dosing schedule possible. It is easier to take a pill once a day than four times a day. Another helpful guideline is to discuss with the prescribing physician drugs with side effects that may be used to a therapeutic advantage. For example, an antidepressant with sedating properties may be a better choice for someone with both depression and trouble sleeping. Everyone should seek evaluation for symptoms that are causing distress; some examples include shortness of breath and pain. No one should be expected to suffer from symptoms when effective forms for managing those symptoms exist.

Treatment of Secondary and Existing Conditions

Of course, patients with FTD also have other medical conditions common to their age group, such as cardiovascular disease, diabetes, hypertension, arthritis, and cancer. FTD patients may have trouble describing specific symptoms, so the caregiver and physician must be vigilant and consider the possibility that new behavioral symptoms are medical in origin. Recently, we witnessed a woman with a urinary catheter, whose rhythmic writhing was due to a urinary tract infection, not the advance of her FTD. Similarly, tooth pain can lead to agitation and aggression in a patient who is unable to describe his or her discomfort. Conversely, repeated visits to the bathroom often represent a compulsion that may be relieved by a serotonin-boosting antidepressant and is not another medical illness.

Many FTD patients will develop symptoms of Parkinson's disease or amyotrophic lateral sclerosis (ALS)—Lou Gehrig's disease. The addition of Parkinsonian symptoms can make the patient prone to falls, and loss of insight into this deficit is particularly problematic with FTD. Patients whose voices weaken or who begin to develop problems with swallowing may be manifesting early symptoms of ALS. When either deficits of movement or ALS occur, life expectancy is markedly diminished and goals and expectations need to be reconsidered.

Medications, particularly SSRIs (Selective Serotonin Reuptake Inhibitors) are often helpful for the FTD patient, as discussed in chapter 5. Because of the vulnerability of FTD patients to Parkinsonian symptoms or ALS, it is important to realize that traditional antipsychotic medications such as chlorpromazine or haloperidol can have devastating effects on the FTD patient. Even the atypical antipsychotic medications such as Zyprexa and Risperdal can exacerbate swallowing deficits. This increases the need to use tiny doses of medications. In addition, we have found that Ritalin can precipitate confusion and agitation. It is often the caregiver who is left with monitoring the different treatments recommended by various specialists.

Participating in Research

There is still so much to learn about FTD. Continued and expanded research is needed regarding causes, prevention, medication management, nonpharmacologic methods for managing behavioral problems, as well as the needs of, and effects on, family members providing care to loved ones with FTD. Ideally, it is best to discuss one's interest in research early in the disease. Each opportunity for participation in research projects must be thoughtfully considered, weighing the risks and benefits for all involved. Participating in a research study should be considered as long as it is not unduly burdensome for the patient and family. Participation in research is often personally rewarding as well as significantly beneficial to future generations. (For more information, see chapters 5, 8, and 9.)

SUMMARY

Caregiving is admirable and rewarding. We hope this chapter has provided some general guidelines to support your efforts throughout the course of this disease as you make multiple, thoughtful decisions with your loved one's health and your own health in mind. The golden rule is to keep the patient's wishes in mind and give yourself permission to reassess the situation. Tough decisions you felt were clearly set may need to be modified when the actual time comes, based on the circumstances faced at that time. Use the support of friends and professionals and base your decisions on your shared beliefs and an organized and focused system of decision making.

CHAPTER 17

Final Choices:

Coping with End-of-Life Concerns

JEANNETTE CASTELLANE

End-of-life concerns affect each of us at some point. Whether we are caring for a spouse, parent, grandparent, or child, we are faced with making decisions that are difficult and challenging. Many of the concerns that will be faced are addressed in this chapter, including carrying out the medical wishes of our loved one, the place where they will be cared for during their last days of life, and the ethics of choosing life-sustaining measures. Specific topics will include the importance of a power of attorney; living wills and advance directives; the impact of nursing homes, hospitals, and hospice; the intervention of CPR; tube feeding; and treatment of secondary illnesses.

The following pages will give you information and hopefully assistance in making these decisions. Caregiving is difficult but caregiving for a person with frontotemporal dementia presents dilemmas many of us have never encountered before.

INSTITUTIONAL VERSUS HOME CARE

Types of Institutional Care

Persons in the later stages of FTD are usually admitted to a hospital because of another acute condition like a fractured hip, urinary tract infection, dehydration, or pneumonia—to name a few conditions. Admission to a hospital is anxiety-causing under normal conditions. A person with a dementia may find it a terrifying experience. The patient may not understand where they are, what is being done to them, and who all the unfamiliar people are that are probing and examining them. In their confusion, individuals may strike out at the staff by trying to bite, kick, or punch them. In this state of fright and combativeness, the patient may try to pull out intravenous lines, catheters, or to climb out of bed. Restraints, both physical and chemical, are sometimes used to subdue the patient. However, utilizing these methods only adds to the confusion.

Families find it upsetting to visit their loved one and see them more confused than when they were in a familiar environment. Once a diagnosis is made and a course of treatment is implemented, the hospital is usually ready to discharge the dementia patient. Hospitals are not experts in treating patients with a dementia. With the geriatric population on the rise, hospitals are beginning to educate their staffs on special needs. They are beginning to understand that a dementia patient needs plenty of tender, loving care and patience. Patients may need one-on-one staffing to keep them calm and reassured. Most hospitals don't have the time or staff available to do this. If the family has financial resources available for private duty care, it may be a short-term solution until discharge.

Once a patient is stabilized, the caseworker will talk in further detail to the family or the nursing home about discharge (if the patient has come to the hospital from a nursing home). From the first day in the hospital, discharge plans should begin. If the family has been taking care of the patient at home, this is the time to seriously think about nursing home placement or help at home. Home healthcare can provide a homemaker or personal care aide. The caseworker should be able to provide assistance with locating resources. Also, the Alzheimer's Association or the Area Agency on Aging can put you in contact with assistance. Chapters 18 and 20 provide information on professional services and places to get support.

Optimally, the family has been looking into nursing homes during earlier stages of the illness, so they are prepared if one is needed. Visiting various facilities, asking the right questions, and putting the patient's name on a waiting list will help to facilitate placement if and when it is needed. Lack of planning can lead to hasty placement that may not be in the best interests of an individual with special needs. Chapter 19 covers nursing home placement in great detail.

Familiar versus Unfamiliar Environment

A familiar environment provides more stability and emotional well-being. Under normal circumstances, new situations can cause anxiety to a person without a dementia. To a certain extent, we all fear the unknown. To those with FTD, being in new environments can be a frightening and often hostile experience in their minds. This unfamiliar place may produce more anxiety and confusion that may lead to the use of chemical and physical restraints.

A familiar environment causes less anxiety and confusion. Whether the person with dementia is at home or in a nursing home, they are in a familiar environment. They see familiar faces, they have a familiar routine, and most important, they are given unconditional love. There is no need to be frightened. Confusion is reduced and comfort is readily available when a fear arises.

The important thing to remember is that dementia patients need familiarity and continuity. Take one of these things away and you present them with an unfamiliar event that is going to produce anxiety leading to more confusion.

Cost of Care

Any illness is costly. A dementia illness is very costly. With dementia, the family is looking at an illness that may go on for many years.

At the time of diagnosis, it is important to look into the financial assessment of the patient and the spouse or family. Decisions must be made at this time as to what financial resources are available and what are the financial concerns for the future. Refer to chapter 21 for detailed coverage of financial preparation, but here are a few critical things to think about.

Begin by looking into the patient's assets and financial resources. How much does she get from social security, pensions, stocks and dividends, savings accounts, rental property, and any other sources of income?

1. Calculate what it will cost to keep the patient in her home or your home with care or modifications to the home. What are the yearly costs for a nursing home versus being at home?
2. What are the costs for medical care going to be? Will insurance policies help pay for any of these costs?
3. If you need to have help or respite care, what is this going to cost?
4. Do you need help to prepare meals, and what will that cost?
5. Are there any legal fees?
6. If the patient remains in his home, what are the annual taxes?
7. What are additional costs in a nursing home, such as hair care, medications, laundry, etc.?
8. Will there be cars or other types of transportation?
9. What are clothing expenses and other miscellaneous items?

The Internal Revenue Service can assist by explaining tax breaks available for the elderly or disabled and persons caring for a family member with dementia. Here is where a good tax consultant or elder lawyer is worth spending money on. They know what can and cannot be deducted and are familiar with federal and state tax laws. They will help to protect your rights and assets. (See chapter 21 for more information.)

Nursing homes can be very expensive. They can cost up to $50,000 or more a year. Financially, this can bankrupt a middle-income family in a matter of two years. Medicare covers acute care but not long-term care. Some coexisting medical conditions may be covered by Medicare and provide for intensive nursing or rehabilitation. Ask Medicare if any condition your loved one has will be covered. Some insurance policies will also cover nursing home costs but they may exclude people with a dementia. The Veterans Administration may also extend benefits to veterans.

Once a person has exhausted their financial resources, he or she eligible to apply for Medicaid. A social worker and the business manager of the nursing home can assist you in applying for Medicaid. The Area Agency on Aging is also a good resource.

At-Home Care

Some families decide that they wish to care for their loved one at home until death occurs. Families come to this decision for any number of reasons, some of which follow.

1. The family may feel strongly that they can give better care than an institution. They know their loved one's habits and needs better than anyone else. The person with dementia may not be able to communicate, but seeing a familiar face and being in a familiar environment is reassuring and calming to them.
2. Some spouses or partners feel that the marriage vows they took or promises they made to care for each other in sickness and health mean just that. They may have made a promise to their loved one never to put them in a nursing home. Breaking that promise may cause them to have considerable guilt.
3. Some cultures expect the family to care for their loved one at home until death occurs. It is expected that members of the close-knit family will help with the care.
4. Some caregivers feel that caring for someone else is the most meaningful thing they can do. They are not looking for praise. They are doing this out of love and respect for the individual. You could almost say it is a vocation for them.

Some things to consider when making this decision are:

1. Make sure you have thoroughly discussed your decision to keep your loved one at home with family, doctor, clergy, and other important people in your life.
2. Thoroughly understand the disease process and what to expect as the disease progresses.
3. Know what resources are available in the community should you need them.
4. Be aware of how the stress of caregiving may impact you physically, mentally, and socially.

Whatever your reason may be, caring for a loved one at home is certainly an option.

HOSPICE CARE

Hospice is not a new concept in modern society. It had its roots back in medieval times when it was a shelter for sick or weary travelers traveling great distances. The basis for hospice, as we know it today, originated in London. In 1967, Dr. Cicely Saunders founded St. Christopher's Hospice to care for dying patients. This concept spread to the United States, and the first state to embrace hospice was Connecticut. Gradually, hospice caught on and it can be found in many different settings throughout our country and the rest of the world.

Many people associate hospice with cancer. This is because many people dying from cancer turn to hospice. However, hospice is applied to all terminal illnesses with a diagnosis of six months or less to live. Hospice is palliative care, emphasizing compassionate care and management of pain and other symptoms. Hospice focuses on quality of life rather than prolonging life. Hospice can be utilized in a hospital setting, in nursing homes, in special hospice inpatient facilities, and in the patient's home.

The hospice concept embraces not only the patient, but the family as well. A specialized team of professionals trained in the hospice philosophy are available to meet the patient's needs and the needs of the family. Involved on the team are trained volunteers, nurses, doctors, aides, clergy, and social workers. Other support personnel, such as a physical therapist or an occupational therapist, may be called in if needed.

Anyone covered by Medicare Part A is eligible for hospice coverage. For the Medicare hospice services to be utilized, the patient must meet three conditions:

1. The physician and the hospice medical director certify that the patient is terminally ill and is expected to live six months or less.
2. The patient or surrogate chooses to use hospice instead of the standard Medicare benefits.
3. The hospice care must be given by a hospice certified by Medicare.

Medicare divides its costs into benefit periods. At the end of each period patients are reevaluated to determine if they still meet the criteria. There are two ninety-day periods and one additional thirty-day period. If patients are recertified as terminally ill, they may have an unlimited extension. However, if a patient chooses to stop hospice at any time, he or she forfeits the remaining benefits in that period.

Medicare hospice will not pay for any services or treatments not related to the terminal illness. However, Medicare will help to pay for costs not related to the terminal illness.

For more detailed information about hospice, contact your physician, a hospital, Medicare-certified hospices in your area, the local health department, or call the National Hospice Organization Help Line (800-658-8898), or on the web at www.nho.org.

ETHICS

What Is Ethics?

Webster's Dictionary defines ethics as, "the study of standards of conduct and moral judgment; moral philosophy." As one delves deeper into the meaning of ethics, many different ideas about what ethics is come into play. In dealing with issues at the end of life, caregivers are asked to make decisions on what should be done based on information provided to them by the patient, the physician, their religion, and other codes of ethics shared by the community.

When an ethical question arises, it is called a dilemma. The caregiver, in the absence of a competent patient, is called upon to resolve an issue. In other words, the caregiver, based upon his ethical principles and values, must choose a course of action. This is not an easy task. Family members may not be in total agreement, medical staff may have different opinions, and the institution itself may be opposed to a caregiver's decision. When such dilemmas occur, an ethics committee may be asked to assist in the dilemma.

Ethics committees are purely advisory. They are made up of staff from within the facility as well as people from the community. It is their responsibility to provide other options, explain policies of the facility, review the dilemma with other similar cases, and provide recommendations that may help to resolve the dilemma. *Remember that ethics committees cannot make decisions; they can only advise.* What an ethics committee studies about the dilemma, and what the committee recommends to the caregiver, is always confidential.

How does a caregiver reach a decision at the end of life? In Hank Dunn's book, *Hard Choices for Loving People,* he asks four questions to help make this decision. These are:

1. *What does the patient want?* This answer can be found in the advance directive, talking with family and friends, and remembering what the patient may have said in a conversation regarding a feeding tube, CPR, etc.
2. *What is in the best interest of the patient?* It is a question of values to keep the patient alive at all costs versus allowing her to die.
3. *What are the prognosis and probable consequences if a certain treatment plan is followed?* The physician needs to discuss all the pros and cons of the treatment. Maybe death with dignity is a better option than treating a condition that may allow the patient to live longer, but will not help him to respond to his environment.
4. *Can I let go?* This is a difficult question for the caregiver. We all want to keep our loved ones around, even though we know their condition is going to get worse. Keep in mind at all times what the patient would have wanted under these circumstances. It is normal to feel guilt and it is difficult to make some tough decisions at the end of life. However, once the decision is made, remember you made it after exploring other options and asking many questions. You have made the right decision for the dilemma as it was presented to you.

Prolonging Life versus Allowing the Disease to Take Its Natural Course.

There comes a point in a person's life when the question arises whether a treatment should be started or ended, or if the person should be allowed to die. This question is made easier if the person has a durable power of attorney for healthcare. Many people do not have these documents. Having a living will and/or a medical durable power of attorney for healthcare decision making is crucial. (See chapter 21 for more information.)

A durable power of attorney for healthcare makes it so much easier for a family to reach a consensus when a loved one is unable to speak for herself. Knowing her wishes and recollecting conversations when she was able to discuss what she wanted eases the decisions at hand. It can be difficult for families to remember that the decision being made is what the patient wants and not what the family may want. It is very hard for loved ones to let go, but they must remember at all times what the patient would want if she were able to make a choice.

When a patient does not have a durable power of attorney for healthcare, it is possible for the court to appoint a legal guardian. This guardian is now the patient's voice in making decisions for care. The guardian should know the patient well enough to make a decision in accordance with what the patient's values and wishes would be.

Whether a guardian is making treatment choices or a durable power of attorney for medical care is in place, the person making the decision must always weigh the benefits and burdens of a particular treatment. What does the advance directive say, what were conversations that the patient had with the decision maker over the years, and what kind of choices had the patient made throughout his life?

Questions to ask about a treatment are:

1. Will this treatment cure the illness? In other words, will the pneumonia be cured but the dementia remain the same?
2. Will the treatment be free of discomfort or pain or more confusion?
3. Will the patient understand enough to allow the treatment to be initiated and continued?
4. If I, as the proxy decision maker, answer no to all the above questions, am I ready to let the illness progress its natural course and let the patient die?

From the time of the diagnosis through the progression of the illness, loved ones consciously or unconsciously have been saying their good-byes as the patient gradually becomes someone they no longer know. *Remember, the decision being made is what the patient would have wanted, not what the decision maker would want.*

What the Patient Would Have Wanted

You will find that during the gradual decline of someone with FTD, you will be called upon over and over again to make difficult decisions. Each change of condition must be made keeping in mind what the patient would have wanted. How do you go about this?

1. Discuss all questions with the patient's physician and medical providers.
2. Ask them if intervention will return the patient to a previous level of care.
3. How long will the intervention delay the progression of the illness?
4. Are there alternative treatments?
5. Discuss all options with the family before making a decision.
6. Remember to do what the patient would have wanted and not what the family would want.

There comes a time when the decision must be made to let the patient go. This is morally and ethically right. It is a difficult decision to make, but it is one that must be made.

FINAL CHOICES

Hospitalization and Medical Intervention

Usually, dementia patients are hospitalized for an illness that cannot be taken care of at home or in a nursing facility. Illness is treated aggressively in a hospital setting. Hospitalization is to cure or make better an illness, and hospitals are required to provide certain life-sustaining procedures. In the case of a person with FTD, we are asking "do we want to prolong his life or do we want to preserve his dignity and enhance what little quality of life he may have left?"

Do you want to hospitalize someone for elective surgery, for example, a bowel obstruction? The caregiver must talk this over with the physician. Sometimes the patient must go to the hospital for her pain needs and treatment cannot be met at home or in the nursing home. This is the time to seriously think about hospice. Again, the caregiver must weight the option of benefits versus burdens.

Treatment Withdrawal and Refusal

Many caregivers, as well as healthcare providers, feel that to withdraw a treatment is to cause the death of the patient. What must be remembered is that the patient has an underlying disease that is causing his body to slowly die. Whether the treatment has begun or is being withdrawn, this underlying disease is going to prove fatal.

Treatments will not work the same way for everyone. Other medical conditions may make it inadvisable to consider a treatment. If a treatment is useless, there is no moral obligation to begin it. One must weigh the benefits and burdens of all treatments. Each case must be decided on its own merits. Again, if it is unknown whether a treatment will be beneficial, try it out for a designated period of time. If it is not beneficial, then it may be withdrawn.

Whatever decision is made regarding withdrawal or refusal of treatment, the emphasis should be placed on making the patient comfortable and allowing her to have a peaceful death.

CPR or Cardiopulmonary Resuscitation

In working with patients and families on a daily basis, the issue of CPR can be controversial. Most cognitively intact patients will say no to CPR: "When my time is up just let me go." Loved ones get upset hearing this, since they don't want to let go. Some will try to persuade their loved one to change his mind, while others will give in to the patient's decision. With an FTD patient, the advance directive can supply the answer.

What happens when there is no advance directive and the patient has never discussed CPR? Begin by asking what CPR is and how it is administered. CPR involves very aggressive chest compression that in all probability will cause fractured ribs, a punctured lung, and perhaps other physical damage. Continue to ask whether the patient will derive any meaningful benefit from having CPR initiated. If CPR is initiated and is successful, will the quality of life be improved for the patient? Are we doing CPR for the caregiver's benefit or because we think the patient, even with an advanced dementia, would have wanted it? CPR may prolong survival by keeping the patient alive on a respirator. Is this the peaceful death the patient may have wanted?

When a person is admitted to a hospital or a nursing home, the question is always asked: Do you want CPR? If CPR is not wanted, make sure the physician writes "No CPR" in the patient's chart, or CPR will be initiated.

Artificial Hydration and Nutrition

This is probably one of most controversial ethical dilemmas. Food and water are the mainstays of our existence. When a person is dying, society still believes everything must be done to maintain nourishment and hydration. Caregivers must be educated that as the body shuts down its systems, it is also providing a relatively comfortable dying process. Sometimes what we decide to do to prolong a life is only creating more distress for the dying patient.

Ethically, using feeding tubes to keep someone alive over a long period of time becomes very controversial. However, in ethics, we discuss benefits versus burdens. In making a decision in any ethical issue one must weigh these benefits and burdens. Ask the physician what some of the benefits of a feeding tube would be and what some of the burdens are. Again, go back to what the patient would have wanted. Would she prefer to be kept alive at all costs, even if it may mean great discomfort and increased risk for infection, leading to other medical problems? Or does the patient prefer to die naturally in relative comfort?

In deciding what to do for a person with late-stage dementia, remember that she doesn't understand what is happening to her. Tube feedings can be invasive and frightening. They may increase her agitation, causing her to pull out the tube. To counteract this, both physical and chemical restraints may be used. This is not the way most people would choose to end their life, suffering from indignity and emotional distress.

Psychologically, tube feedings take away the human touch. A person responds to touch and love. Personal interaction is lost with tube feeding. Swallowing difficulties are the end stage of dementia. It is difficult to make the decision to consent to tube feeding or not. Some caregivers have opted to use a feeding tube on a trial basis. They agree to try for a certain period of time. If the patient has not shown improvement or has become agitated over the use of a feeding tube, it will be removed. This sometimes helps to lessen the guilt the caregiver may be having about the decision.

Perhaps Hank Dunn sums up the question of a feeding tube best. He says, "Unless the patient has given specific instructions preferring a feeding tube, I believe artificial feeding of those with Alzheimer's disease or other dementias is a totally inappropriate treatment. It does not cure the underlying disease, it does not prevent death, it does not even offer a longer life than for those who do not receive a tube, and the numerous burdens of a feeding tube for these patients are not counterbalanced by any benefit."

Letting Go

All of our life we have had to make decisions. Some of our decisions have been good and others have failed. From the time we are able to decide what is right and what is wrong, we are making decisions. Our parents gave us the groundwork to make decisions. It was difficult for our parents to "let go" when we stepped inside of school for the first time. From then on we had many more "let go"s. We left our childhood behind and became adults with added responsibilities. Parents age and start to look to us for guidance. The roles begin to reverse.

It is natural for us to not want to let go of someone we love. However, there comes a time when a decision must be made to let go of a loved one who is suffering from a terminal illness. How we handle this decision will depend on how we have faced difficult times before. We look to our spiritual self and how we face our own mortality. Are we able to say to our loved one, "I love you but now I must let you go"? We cannot stop death but we can learn to accept it no matter how painful it may be.

Families of people with a dementia slowly let go, starting at the time of diagnosis. It is a slow and painful experience to see our loved ones change before our eyes. Without realizing it, the caregiver has been going through the dying process and letting go all along the way.

Are you ready to let go? If we are honest with ourselves, the answer would probably be no. However, there comes a time to let go. Remember the good times you had and don't dwell on what the disease has done to your loved one. You have done the best you know how.

BIBLIOGRAPHY

Dunn, H. *Hard Choices for Loving People: CPR, Artificial Feeding, Comfort Measures Only, and the Elderly Patient*, 3d ed. Herndon, Va.: A and A Publishers, 1994.

Idziak, J. *Ethical Dilemmas in Long-Term Care*, study ed. Simon and Kolz Publishing, 2000.

Mace, N., and P. Rabins. *The 36-Hour Day*, rev. ed. Baltimore, Md.: Johns Hopkins University Press, 1991.

National Hospice Organization. *Hospice Under Medicare.* South Deerfield, Mass.: Channing L. Bete, 1997.

Post, A. *The Moral Challenge of Alzheimer's Disease*, 2d ed. Baltimore, Md.: Johns Hopkins University Press, 2000.

Webster's New World Dictionary of the American Language, 3d college ed. New York: Simon and Schuster, 1988.

Part III
Caregiver Resources

CHAPTER 18

Professional Caregiving:
Using Health Community Services

JUDY L. FISHER AND SUSAN RILEY

Professional caregiving comes in a variety of dimensions and facets, allowing the healthcare consumer a menu of options from which to select. Along with the aforementioned services are the much-sought-after funding sources by which professional caregiving may be reimbursed. The objective of this chapter is to provide the knowledge necessary to pursue excellence in health care for loved ones.

HOME HEALTH CARE

Home health care can be defined as a component of a continuum of comprehensive health care, whereby health services are provided to individuals and families in their place of residence for the purpose of promoting, maintaining, or restoring health, or of maximizing the level of independence while minimizing illness. Services appropriate to the needs of the individual patient and family are planned, coordinated, and made available by providers organized for the delivery of home care through the use of employed staff, contractual arrangements, or a combination of the two patterns.

A home healthcare agency is known as "certified" when specific federal and state criteria are met in order for the agency to be deemed qualified to provide Medicare (federally funded health insurance) and/or Medicaid (state-funded health insurance) reimbursed services to persons residing at home.

A "noncertified" home healthcare agency is an agency that usually provides services similar to that of a certified home healthcare agency, yet with different funding sources. Some noncertified agencies are eligible to provide services reimbursed by specific state-funded programs.

Both certified and noncertified home healthcare agencies usually are licensed by the state in which they are located and are eligible to provide services reimbursed by private insurance companies when specific criteria are met. Most private insurance companies, including managed-care companies, require a home healthcare agency to be accredited by a nationally recognized accrediting organization, such as the Joint Commission on Accreditation of Healthcare Organizations.

Home Health Personnel

Home healthcare personnel come in a variety of disciplines and have specific goals as defined by a physician's plan of care or a plan established by the family. The most common disciplines to provide home healthcare services are registered nurses, licensed practical/vocational nurses, physical therapists, occupational therapists, speech pathologists, social workers, home health aides, companions/homemakers, and twenty-four-hour live-in caregivers.

Registered nurses are clinicians who provide direct nursing care and ongoing assessment of patients and families. They are educators because they teach patients and families how to care for themselves and one another. The licensed practical/vocational nurse works directly under the auspice of the registered nurse. Both must be licensed by the state in which they practice.

Speech pathologists work with people with a communication problem related to speech, language, cognition, or hearing. Speech pathologists also work with persons with eating or swallowing problems. (See chapter 10 for more information.)

Physical therapists provide maintenance, preventive, and restorative treatment for patients in the home. Activities include strengthening muscles, restoring mobility, controlling spasticity, gait training, and teaching active-passive resistive exercises. (See chapter 11 for more information.)

Occupational therapists help patients achieve their optimum level of functioning by teaching them to develop and maintain the abilitiy to perform activities of daily living in their home. (See chapters 12, 13, and 14 for more information.)

Social workers in home health care hold a master's degree in social work and help patients and families deal with social, emotional, and environmental factors that affect their well-being. Social workers assist directly in intervening or referring patients to appropriate community resources. Often, after an episode in the hospital, patients return home unable to cope with their present state of functioning and require assistance in adjusting to their functional limitations.

*Home health aide*s are directly supervised by the home healthcare nurse or therapist. The role of the home health aide is to help patients reach their optimal level of independence by temporarily assisting with personal hygiene as well as light housekeeping duties and other homemaking skills. The home health aide must be experienced as an aide and trained as a certified home health aide if they are to provide and direct hands-on patient care.

Companion service is provided to persons needing only supervision and/or light housekeeping and meal preparation. Companions may run errands such as grocery shopping, picking up prescriptions, etc. Medicare and some Medicaid programs do not reimburse this service and employees should be bonded.

Twenty-four-hour live-in service is provided to persons requiring or desiring a caregiver to live in their home to provide care or companionship. These caregivers are trained in housekeeping, meal preparation, and may run errands. Medicare or Medicaid does not reimburse this service and employees should be bonded.

Knowing When to Use Professional Services

This decision is very individualized. Some families are able to pull together enough formal and informal support among the family members and/or friends and neighbors. It is important for one to recognize when stress and burn-out have taken their toll. When caregiving becomes your sole defining role you may want to consider the services of professionals. Caregivers need to maintain their own identity outside of this role and have some personal time, independent of the patient.

Primary Management of Services

If the services being provided are certified services, the agency providing the services will have a case/care manager on staff. For other services, one can look to hire a care manager on a private pay basis or look to governmental agencies such as an agency on aging or for the disabled.

Precertification, Services, and Payment

The insurance carrier will determine what services, if any, are authorized. For traditional fee-for-service Medicare and Medicaid, agencies will provide services in accordance with the respective established guidelines and criteria.

Timeline of Therapies and Services

The duration of services/therapies is dependent upon many variables such as the type of insurance, diagnosis, prognosis, rate of progress, and medical and financial need. Services are individualized as prescribed in the plan of care. Those paying privately for services can continue indefinitely. Generally, therapies end when an individual reaches a goal or plateaus. In the case of managed care, therapy generally ends when the insurance company no longer approves it.

Getting Aides in the Home While Receiving Therapy

With managed care, it would depend on whether or not the insurance will approve it. With traditional Medicare it is possible; however, it depends on the diagnosis and the reason for therapy, along with the reason for the ADL deficit. Medicaid programs generally cover this service but this too may vary from state to state.

ADULT DAYCARE CENTERS

Health-oriented daycare centers provide health and physical rehabilitation, whereas multipurpose daycare centers provide social activities and interaction. Daycare centers serve the person who has some physical or mental limitation that interferes with totally independent living and who needs social, nutritional, or recreational services. Daycare centers also allow the permanent caretaker to use day hours for work or other activities. Daycare centers are a viable alternative to institutionalization.

Funding for daycare centers is available through some private insurance and managed-care organizations as well as other sources. Research what funding is available with the specific daycare center.

Choosing a Facility

When choosing a facility it is important to visit first, unannounced if possible. There should be an R.N. available at all times when clients are present. Other important factors to consider are staff-to-client ratio, security features (i.e., alarm systems to protect clients), and staff attitude toward caregiving. Check to see that there is a full calendar of activities for the clients and ascertain that therapeutic activities are based on the client's diagnosis and/or disability.

Considering Staff Type, Staff-to-Client Ratio, and Numbers of People Attending

Daycare facilities in different states may have different requirements for types of staff and staff-to-client ratios. Generally speaking, the more clients the more staff. It is best to visit and observe. Ask the facility staff what the ratio is and what the requirements are, if any. For example, in the state of New Jersey the standard R.N.-to-client ratio is 1:60 and direct, full-time, equivalent-care attendants is 1:9.

State/County versus Private Facilities

If a daycare receives government funding, it is likely that there will be a set of standards that the daycare must meet in order to continue to receive that funding. Private facilities may not have to meet the same standards, but they are permitted to exceed them.

Criteria for Attending Medical Daycare

To attend a medical daycare one must have a medical diagnosis. Psychiatric diagnoses alone do not permit admission. Private facilities may admit whomever they choose, regardless of diagnosis. Generally, a government-funded facility will have criteria that must be met, one of which includes a diagnosis that warrants medical daycare. Every daycare has different criteria. For some, patients must be ambulatory, for others they may have to be continent, or able to feed themselves. It is best to check directly with the facility.

FUNDING SOURCES FOR SERVICES

Medicare

Reimbursement of home health services is handled through insurance companies that are under contract with the Social Security Administration to pay home healthcare agencies for Medicare-covered services rendered to beneficiaries. To qualify for home health services, a beneficiary must be sixty-five years of age or disabled, and under the care of a physician; meet the homebound criteria; or in need of skilled nursing services, physical therapy, occupational therapy, or speech therapy on an intermittent basis. Skilled services are those required by an individual that are reasonable and necessary for treatment of an illness or injury.

Medicaid

Authorized by Title XIX of the Social Security Act, Medicaid provides health services to low-income persons. It is a medical assistance program for eligible people under Aid to Families with Dependent Children or Supplemental Security Income of the Social Security Act and also is available for those individuals whose income is insufficient to cover medical services and for disability coverage. Medicaid is administered by the states but is both state and federally subsidized. Medicaid covers home health, including skilled and unskilled services such as personal care.

Private Insurance

Third-party payers are represented by private insurance companies to which the person subscribes individually or with a group such as an employer. Some states have laws that require home health to be a provision in health insurance coverage. Individuals under sixty-five years of age who need home care follow-up after surgery or prolonged hospitalization use this benefit the most.

Private Pay

Some individuals who require home health services but do not have health insurance may pay the home health agency directly. Individuals who do not meet their insurance coverage requirements and still want the services pay the established charge or may be offered the service on a sliding scale or established fee, based on their financial status.

State Agencies on Aging

The federal government, through the Department of Health and Human Services, and the Administration on Aging, direct funding specifically to assist the aging population to remain independent in their homes. The Administration on Aging is divided into ten different regions. Each state within the regions has its own branch, division, or agency. Funds may be used differently by each state and the amounts they receive also may vary. However, there are some target areas, such as nutrition and home assistance services, that are just about universal. All state aging offices can provide information and referral services to assist you in your journey seeking professional caregiving services. If you know your local department, it would likely be easier to begin there rather than at the state level.

State Agencies on the Disabled

State offices on disability services are quite different. While each state does have a Division of Developmental Disabilities that receives federal funding, only a handful of states have the state level divisions or offices of disability services that are generic and have a cross-disability focus. The best way to begin is to see if your state has such a division; if so, contact the one in your local area and see what services are offered.

State Offices on Mental Health

Mental health services also may be available in your community. The easiest way to find services of this nature is to contact your state Department of Mental Health and ask to be directed to mental health services and providers serving your area. What is available will vary by state and community.

Veterans Administration

The Veterans Administration offers various types of assistance, including but not limited to medications, nursing home care, hospitalization, and respite care. Services offered may differ by state. To find out what is available in your area, contact your local or state Veteran's Administration office.

Grant Funding

Frequently, specific services are available through grants. A provider agency may have their own grants that they have written and for which they have obtained funding. Other monies can be obtained from state and federal funds that are distributed through a request for proposal, or RFP. Here, specific agencies apply to receive funds to provide direct service. Home healthcare providers, if nonprofit, are generally able to provide some service through some form of grant funding. Funding obtained through the Older Americans Act is one source example.

Private Foundations

Private foundations are another avenue to pursue. Special-interest groups may be able to help, such as disability-specific groups. This type of funding is a little more difficult to obtain and requires a bit of research and networking.

CHAPTER 19

Home Away from Home:

Nursing Home and Assisted-Living Options

MORRIS J. KAPLAN

WHEN A NURSING HOME IS NECESSARY; FINDING A GOOD ONE

Deciding whether to place a loved one in a nursing home can be one of the most difficult decisions a caregiver can face. The mere thought can arouse overwhelming feelings of guilt, failure, hopelessness, and fear. This chapter will provide a framework for a caregiver to examine objectively whether nursing home placement is in the best interest of a loved one with dementia. This is followed by a discussion of how to find a good nursing home, exactly what to look for, and a description of some of the programs found at facilities that have adopted *best care practices.*

Excellent care can most often be provided at home. However, certain conditions and situations can arise over the course of a neurodegenerative illness that suggest additional interventions are needed to ensure a person's highest level of functioning and comfort. Key areas of concern are weight loss, skin ulcers, over/under-medication, incontinence, and personal safety. When problems arise in these areas, the caregiver needs to determine where corrective interventions can be effectively implemented either at home or in a nursing facility that has adopted best care practices.

KEY DETERMINING FACTORS

Significant weight loss (5 percent in the last 30 days or 10 percent in the last 180 days) is something that needs to be addressed and corrected. Significant weight loss is not a normal part of a dementia illness until the very end stage of life. Interventions such as special high-calorie and high-protein foods and supplements, together with specialized feeding assistance programs and techniques, can and should be instituted to reverse the weight loss and maintain adequate nutrition and hydration. Weight loss should be seen by the caregiver as an avoidable condition. The caregiver needs to determine whether the interventions can be implemented at home.

Pressure ulcers (bedsores) are not a normal part of aging. Good toileting care, incontinence care, skin care, nutrition, and proper positioning should prevent most pressure ulcers except in the end stages of the disease. Persistent reddened areas on the skin indicate an immediate high risk for sores. Preventative skin care, nutritional interventions, and pressure relieving interventions (discussed later in the chapter) should be an integral part of the ongoing care program. When a pressure ulcer develops, the interventions must be intensified and skillfully implemented to heal the wound. Presence of pressure ulcers is often a significant indicator of *avoidable* decline in health. It should be acknowledged by the caregiver as a signal that action must be taken either at home or in an appropriately capable nursing facility.

Over/under medicating is another avoidable and common condition among persons with dementia. Overmedication promotes falls, lethargy, and major decline in activities of daily living. Often, psychotropic drugs are used or misused to lessen behavioral symptoms. At home, caregivers may find little alternative to dispensing a "calming" medication to allow for some respite or sleep for the caregiver and patient. Signs of unsteady gait, lethargy, and/or an acute decrease in verbal, cognitive, and functional abilities may be caused by medication use and represent a serious problem. Much literature suggests that the use of nine or more different medications greatly increases the risk of adverse reactions. If the number of medications exceeds nine, or if any of the signs of overmedication are present, the caregiver should take this as a sign that corrective action may be needed and if such action can be taken at home. Alternatively, a good facility will have nurses and an involved geriatric psychiatrist who have experience in identifying and correcting instances of over-medication.

Incontinence will likely occur in the middle or later stages of a dementia. The onset of incontinence can often be delayed. A few of the critical interventions in delaying the onset of incontinence include: not using any kind of physical restraint; providing appropriate prompting; cueing and cueing aids; providing regular, scheduled physical assistance to, and on, the toilet; maintaining ambulation and range of motion in the extremities through restorative exercise programs; and avoiding overmedication. The preservation of bowel and bladder continence should be an ongoing, closely monitored goal of the caregiver. The primary caregiver should assess whether these interventions are being provided at home. If they are not, consideration should be given to identifying an appropriately capable nursing facility.

Personal safety is an important consideration. If a person wanders or easily gets lost when leaving the home, special automatic door locking devices (that disengage in case of fire) may be needed. Becoming lost outside the home can not only traumatize the person with FTD and the caregiver, it can also lead to serious injury. If this does happen, the caregiver should either equip the home with an effective egress restricting system (e.g., Wanderguard) or consider placement in a facility that is properly equipped.

A caregiver must also consider safety inside the home. Access to dangerous items such as poisonous liquids, sharp knives and instruments, matches, etc. should be restricted. (See chapter 14 for more information.) If there has been any incidence of unsafe use of appliances, especially in the kitchen, the caregiver must take steps to prevent catastrophes like fire. The caregiver should consider a safe facility if the home cannot be made safe for the person with dementia.

Often, a caregiver's response to wandering, abusive behavior, or frequent falling is to physically restrain the patient. Physical restraint is dangerous and can lead to serious injury or death. In addition, there is nothing more effective in promoting incontinence, overall physical decline, mood and psychosocial decline, despair, fear, and agitation than tying a person down. There are safe and effective alternatives to physically restraining a person (a discussion of which is beyond the scope of this chapter). If the caregiver has resorted to tying down the person with dementia (with a seat belt, a tied vest, a lap tray, lap cushion, roller bar, two siderails in bed, etc.), that caregiver should consider placement in a facility that is restraint-free.

Certainly, treatment such as wound care, tube feeding, administration of IV medications, and rehabilitation therapy all indicate that skilled nursing or rehab care must be provided. This can be done either by bringing in professional nurses or therapists from home care agencies or by finding, even temporarily, placement in a facility.

If after considering the issues of weight loss, skin ulcers, overmedication, incontinence, and personal safety, a caregiver has concluded that interventions are needed that cannot be provided in the home, the caregiver's next task is to identify a facility where *best care practices* have been successfully implemented. Finding a nursing facility where these methods have been adopted requires careful research. The next section will identify essential sources of information and how to use them.

SOURCES OF INFORMATION

A starting point is the local area agency on aging and the office of the ombudsman in the county in which you live or nearby county. You can find the Area Agency on Aging in the phone book. The agency can provide you with a list of nursing homes in the county. The ombudsman, usually a part of the agency, is the person who represents nursing home residents and their families in addressing problems at nursing homes. The ombudsman can be an invaluable resource in steering you (probably "off the record") toward or away from certain facilities. If the ombudsman is not forthcoming, ask which facilities he or she regularly is called upon to visit.

The local chapter of the Alzheimer's Association can be a valuable resource in identifying good nursing facilities. The association office may direct you to individuals who have personal experience with certain facilities or to local caregiver support groups. The people in support groups often have loved ones in facilities and can give you first-hand information about them. *There is no better source of information about a facility than the family of a resident.* Another very valuable resource is the National Citizen's Coalition for Nursing Home Reform (NCCNHR).[1] NCCNHR is a very vocal and effective national organization that advocates for the rights of nursing home residents. NCCNHR will direct you to individuals or local advocacy groups in your state who can help steer you in the right direction.

After identifying a number of facilities, the next step is to research the data on each facility provided by the state and federal government. Each nursing home in the country is inspected annually by the state's department of health. The state inspection report or "survey report" must be posted in each facility. It is based on a surveyor's interpretation of the facility's compliance with state and federal regulations. Unfortunately, there is extreme variation in the interpretation of these regulations by surveyors and offices. This results in extreme inconsistency in the quality of survey reports and in enforcement action against nursing homes.

The survey report can be helpful, or it can be misleading. Surveyors are either too easy or too tough. It is often impossible for a consumer to tell the difference. If a sanction has been imposed as a result of the survey (such as a monetary fine, a ban on admissions, a ban on Medicaid or Medicare payments, or a termination of the facility's nursing assistant training program), that should be seen as a dangerous sign that very serious care problems were found. However, the absence of such sanctions does not at all suggest that there are not serious care problems.

So how do you know if a survey report accurately reflects the care? It is very important to use a new tool that the federal government has recently made available—the Facility Quality Indicator Profile or "Quality Indicator (QI) Report." The QI Report focuses on specific objective indicators of quality (or the lack of it). The QI Report looks at twenty-four healthcare characteristics among the nursing home's residents. These twenty-four characteristics or "quality indicators" have been selected by Centers for Medicare and Medicaid Services (CMS, formerly HCFA)[2] as key areas that can show either quality or lack of quality in a nursing home's delivery of care.

The QI Report is updated monthly and is based on data contained in the Minimum Data Set (MDS) assessment form. An MDS is completed by nurses at least quarterly on each resident. The MDS asks hundreds of questions about a resident's health problems and care needs. The most valuable part of the QI Report for consumers is the column titled "Percentile Rank," which shows the percentile ranking of the nursing home relative to all nursing homes in the state. A nursing home is given a percentile rank for each of the twenty-four quality indicators.

A rank in the top third (that is, the 0–33 percentile) on a particular quality indicator is a sign that good care practices are probably present. This should be the consistent score on the majority of at least the nine quality indicators identified below. *The lower the percentile rank, the better.* The quality indicators that are the most revealing about the level of quality at a nursing home are the following:

- #6, the use of nine or more medications.
- #12, prevalence of urinary tract infection. Urinary tract infections can often be the result of inadequate hygiene or incontinence care, inadequate assistance with hydration, and unnecessary use of indwelling catheters.
- #13, the prevalence of weight loss.
- #15 and #11, the prevalence of dehydration or fecal impaction. Both should rarely if ever occur except when near death.
- #17, the incidence of decline in late loss ADLs (activities of daily living). Late loss ADLs include turning in bed, transferring in or out of bed or chair, toileting, and eating.
- #18, the incidence of decline in ROM (range of motion). Good restorative nursing programs and the elimination of physical restraints will lower the incidence of decline in ability to perform ADLs and ROM.
- #22, the use of physical restraints.
- #24, the incidence of pressure ulcers/bedsores.

It is important to note that a percentile ranking that is not in the top third (the 0–33 percentile) in a particular quality indicator does not automatically indicate a failure of the facility to provide good care in that area. It is possible that the indicator ranking reflects conditions or characteristics of residents that developed *prior* to admission to the facility or that may be the result of the end stage of a disease. The caregiver should ask the facility for an explanation about each indicator listed above that falls outside of the 0–33 percentile ranking.

While there are areas where the Quality Indicator Report system can be strengthened, this new tool provides consumers and regulators with tremendously important and unprecedented insight into the quality of a nursing home's delivery of care. *The Quality Indicator Report is one of the most valuable tools for a nursing home consumer.* The QI Report for a facility is only available at the facility. You must ask to see it. If the facility has a good Quality Indicator Report, it is most likely a facility that has successfully implemented best care practices.

The federal government provides some nursing home survey and quality indicator information at CMS's Web site, www.medicare.gov. At that site, click on "Nursing Home Compare." The Nursing Home Compare site is continually being revised by CMS in an attempt to make it more helpful to consumers. Generally, the site includes information on selecting a nursing home and information about any particular nursing home or group of homes in a geographic area. The site contains the summarized results of the most recent state inspection and some of the quality indicator information discussed above. The exact format of the QI information may change from time to time. Generally, it will include, at a minimum, information about the incidence of pressure ulcers (bedsores), restraint use, and weight loss. When you visit the nursing home in person, you should ask to see the full Quality Indicator Report.

It should also be noted that several states have Web sites that provide information on nursing homes. The best way to find the Web address is to either call your state capital building and ask for the department of health or use an Internet search engine like Yahoo (type in the name of the state and either "department of health" or "nursing homes" or "government"). This should direct you to your state's department of health Web site, if there is one. From there, look for any links that deal with nursing homes. The Pennsylvania Department of Health Web site, for example, gives the full text of the several most recent inspection reports for each nursing home.[3] The Maryland Department of Health has a Web site that gives detailed information about each nursing home's Quality Indicator Reports.[4]

VISITING HOMES IN PERSON

After checking the above resources, your next step is visiting the nursing home. You will need to call and schedule an appointment to get a complete tour and information about prices and availability. But you can also make an unannounced visit. This section will identify important things to observe, questions to ask staff and families, and specific care programs to investigate.

When you visit the nursing home, look at the interaction between staff and residents and between staff and you. Is it a friendly and warm place? As you walk through the home, do people greet you and make you feel welcome? Are staff members speaking to residents, holding their hands, hugging them, keeping them company, giving assistance in a caring, compassionate way? Focus more on the way the staff interacts with the residents and less on the elegance of the furnishings.

Are the residents dressed neatly and in clean clothes? Are their fingernails trimmed? Are the men shaved? Are staff members responding to residents who may be calling for help? Is the home clean? Does it smell clean, or is there an unpleasant odor? Is the home a lively place with different activities going on? Are residents involved in group programs? Are people walking or ambulating with wheelchairs freely throughout the building? Or are they physically restrained in some way (a seat belt, a tray or cushion across their wheelchair or a vest restraint)? Are residents confined in bed with two full-length siderails? Do most of the residents appear lethargic and "zombied out"? Do you see many staff, especially at meal time? Are the staff assisting residents (with walking, eating, transferring from place to place)?

One of the first things you want to request from the admissions person is the most recent Quality Indicator Report. Use the guidelines discussed previously to frame your questions. If there is reluctance to share this information with you, ask why and ask to speak to the administrator or director of nursing. If necessary, ask to make an appointment to meet later. If they won't share the Quality Indicator Report with you, realize that your search for a good facility has not yet ended.

Either during or after the tour seek out and speak to staff members. Approach at least two nurses and three nursing assistants and ask them how they like working at the facility and how long they have been there. Ask how the management treats the staff. Ask how often the facility uses "agency staff" (temporary staffing from outside companies). Extensive use of agency staff may suggest problems with adequate staffing and consistency in staffing. Ask if they feel the facility has enough staff (nurses and nursing assistants). Perhaps most important of all, ask a nursing assistant (not the admissions person) how many residents she takes care of and on which shift (day, evening, or night—the number will vary depending on the shift). Take notes and compare them later with the suggested staffing ratios discussed below.

If the staff is happy, treated well by the management, and consists of enough personnel to do the job, chances are the care will be good and the residents will be happy and treated well. The opposite is likely to be true if the staff is unhappy, unstable, and insufficient to do the work.

During a visit to the facility, seek out people who are visiting residents. These are usually family members. They can be found most often during mealtimes. As stated earlier, there is no better source of information about a facility than the family of a resident of the facility. Ask how long their loved one or friend has been at the facility. Ask what they think of the place, the staff, and the management. Ask them whom they go to if they have a problem or need, and ask if their problems or needs get addressed. Ask them if they would recommend the facility for your loved one. Remember, no facility or person is perfect and can please everyone. So always ask more than one family or visitor.

NURSING HOME BEST CARE PRACTICES

Elements of nursing home best care practices for the care of persons with dementia include effective management, adequate staffing, weight loss prevention programs, effective skin care programs, appropriate socialization and cognitive support programs, restraint elimination, staff training programs, and a geriatric psychiatry program. The following section will give a brief introduction to these care programs.

Effective care-plan meetings are one important element of best care practices. It can be extremely valuable, though not common, to observe a care-plan meeting. The care-plan meeting is the periodic meeting where the management team of the facility meets to discuss the condition and care of a resident. To observe a meeting, you would have to make arrangements with the admissions person, who would have to obtain permission from the resident being discussed or the resident's family.

The meeting usually includes the resident's supervisor nurse, the director of nursing, the administrator, the family of the resident, a social worker, activities department staff, and the dietician or dietary department manager. Your task as an observer is to determine how well the team knows the resident, the resident's physical condition and care needs, preferences as far as activities and meals, and major issues regarding the resident's nursing care. If they know the resident well and are interacting and deciding as a group on the resident's plan of care, especially on changes needed to address the resident's condition, they are doing good work. If the key personnel listed above are not even present, and if there is no evidence that anyone really knows the resident, the opposite is probably true.

The most important element of an effective best care practices program is an active leadership committed to a mission of caring and possessing the knowledge of what best care practices are and how to implement them. The second most important element is adequate staffing. In this author's fifteen years of experience, in order to have a happy and motivated staff, happy residents, and consistently outstanding healthcare outcomes as measured by the Quality Indicator Reports, *adequate staffing means a minimum of 3.3 nursing staff hours per resident per day.*[5]

When it comes to staff-to-resident ratios, the most significant number is the number of residents a nursing assistant (separate from the nurses) has to care for. On the first shift, there should be at least one nursing assistant for every eight residents. On the second shift, there should be at least one nursing assistant for every nine residents. On the third shift there should be at least one nursing assistant for every fifteen residents.[6]

The practice of "permanent assignments," where the same nursing assistant is assigned the same residents everyday, is also especially important in the care of residents with dementia. It enables the nursing assistant to learn the resident's particular needs, preferences, and routine. It enables the resident to get to know and feel comfortable with the nursing assistant.

A good weight loss prevention program starts with assistance with eating. The needs of the dementia patient change over time and are very different depending on the stage of the disease—early, middle, or advanced. There should be three distinct dining programs. The first is for high-functioning residents who eat with minimal assistance. The second is geared toward people in the middle stages of dementia. These residents are able to feed themselves but tend to forget to finish eating, get distracted and wander away, or act in inappropriate ways (playing with foods or pushing things off the table). These residents need extensive cueing, step-by-step instruction, directing, and encouragement by staff using a host of assistive techniques. This type of program requires a ratio of one staff member to three residents and lasts for at least ninety minutes. The third program is geared toward people in the late stages of dementia who require extensive to total assistance with eating. *This program requires a ratio of approximately one staff member to 2 to 2$^1/_2$ residents.*

The nutrition program should include the taking of weekly weights for those who have had significant weight loss (5 percent in 30 days or 10 percent in 180 days) as well as monthly dietician evaluations and recommendations. Identifying and accommodating the resident's food preferences is critical. A best practices facility will have a special menu of foods for people with weight loss. Such foods would include gravies, juices, milks, baked goods, hot cereals, mashed potatoes, and other items that are packed with sugar, butter, margarine, cream, half and half, condensed milk, dry milk solids, etc. High-calorie and high-protein supplements, drinks, milkshakes, and snacks should be provided throughout the day and night. Proof of the success of the nutrition and weight loss prevention program can be found in the facility's ranking for weight loss on its Quality Indicator Report.

The skin care program should be multifaceted. Proper hydration, nutrition and weight gain programs, proper vitamin and nutrient intake, good incontinence care, good exercise and range-of-motion programs, regular body repositioning and turning—all of which require adequate staffing—are essential to the avoidance of skin breakdown. Each resident must be assessed on at least a quarterly basis to determine the risk of skin breakdown and to identify necessary preventative measures. If possible, skin breakdown must be recognized and treated at its earliest stage—an unopened, persistent reddened area.

Once a sore is open, a nurse specially trained as a certified Continence Wound Ostomy Care Nurse (CWOCN) or Enterostomal Therapist (ET) needs to be involved. Such a nurse has received special postbachelor's degree (AB) training in wound care and should not be confused with a "treatment nurse" or "wound nurse" who has no such certification. Only a best practices facility will have such certified nurses. In addition to this level of expertise, a best practices facility will have a sufficient number of specialized pressure-relieving mattress systems. The depth of the wound will dictate the type of system to be used. Choices range from high-density foam mattresses to motorized low-air-loss mattresses to motorized alternating pressure mattresses. The motorized mattresses are very expensive but are invaluable tools in curing bedsores, as are a variety of gel and foam cushions for pressure relief in wheelchairs. A facility's arsenal against bedsores will also include pressure relieving pads, cones, pillowlike cushions, and a host of other products. Proof of the success of the facility's skin care program can be found in the facility's ranking for pressure ulcers on its QI Report.

A best practices facility will have activities and socialization programs that seek to maximize psychosocial functioning by providing enriching, nurturing, and satisfying experiences for residents with dementia. As with dining, the psychosocial needs of people with FTD vary significantly over the course of the illness. A facility should offer at least three levels of activity programs, each at least twice daily. The first level should be geared to the nondemented residents, but should include one activity each day that is open to the entire resident community.

The second level should be geared to those in the early and middle stages of a dementia illness. The aim of this level is to maintain and encourage socialization and interaction with others through a variety of ability-appropriate, meaningful, and enjoyable activities. These should be conducted with smaller groups of people who are still verbal and communicative. A skilled program leader, who goes with the flow of the conversation and provides reassurance and affirmation, can do wonders in restoring self-confidence and preserving the skills needed for communication and social interaction.

The third level of programming is for those in the late stages of dementia who are generally immobile and nonverbal. The focus of this programming is remotivation and stimulation. Residents with advanced dementia respond especially well to music. Music therapy, in a variety of forms, together with various sensory stimulation activities, aim to promote an individual's awareness of self and the environment.

A best practices facility will be a restraint-free facility. As you tour the facility, look to see if residents are restrained in chairs with seat belts, barrier cushions, hard trays (like in a baby's high chair) or tied vests. Look also to see if residents in bed are restrained with two full-length side rails. If you see more than one or two residents with such devices, you have not yet found a best practices facility.

A critical element is staff training. Training in dementia care should be provided at the time of orientation and then at least annually. Topics should include how to communicate with people with dementia, how to determine the needs of a confused or nonverbal resident, how to analyze and respond to changes in mood or behavior, how to respond to extreme behavioral symptoms, and how to provide ADL care to a confused or resistive person.

Finally, a best care practices facility will have an involved geriatric psychiatrist. This professional will work closely with the nursing staff to address the psychiatric needs of the residents, particularly depression, and to tailor the use of psychotropic medications so that side effects such as lethargy are avoided.

Conclusion

The caregiver should use the suggested guidelines to identify whether a condition exists that requires care that cannot reasonably be provided at home. If such a condition exists, the caregiver should follow the suggested investigation process to identify whether a best practices facility exists nearby and whether admission is possible. The search for a best practices facility is not necessarily an easy one. Doing the research, seeking referrals, looking for the important signs, asking the right questions, all take time and effort. But while so much of the dementia disease is beyond the caregiver's control, the tools outlined above can empower the caregiver and put him or her back in control.

ASSISTED LIVING

For people in the early and middle stages of dementia, and their families, an assisted-living facility can provide a secure and beneficial environment. A good facility can be a safe haven that can help a person maintain his or her highest practical level of independence, socialization, and well-being. In general, it will provide physical safety and security, socialization, companionship and meaningful activity, and assistance with activities of daily living. There is, however, significant variation in the scope of programming and services provided by facilities. Since FTD entails a progressive decline over time in cognitive, self-care, and physical abilities, it is very important to understand the scope of services provided by a particular facility. If the caregiver understands limits of services, and monitors for changes and declines in an individual's condition that may trigger the need for a different care setting, an assisted-living facility can be a valuable and therapeutic option.

For those in the early stages of FTD, it is important to maintain physical safety. The home in which they lived safely may now present opportunities for injury. Working safely with knives and appliances may be an insurmountable challenge for the formerly expert chef or homemaker. A walk or drive to a nearby store or friend's house may result in an unintended journey far off course.

A good assisted-living facility for the cognitively impaired provides a safe environment that is tailored to the needs and limitations of the person with dementia. A good facility will have:

- a continuous indoor walking or wandering circuit and an enclosed outdoor courtyard or garden
- an automatic door-locking system that prevents unescorted egress
- special bracelets worn by residents that will trigger the exit doors to lock, except in case of a fire emergency
- a centrally located residential style kitchen with all the makings of a home kitchen, equipped with special safety features (switches and locks, etc.) that restrict the use of sharp items and cooking appliances so that they can only be used with the supervision of a staff member
- a conveniently located residential style laundry room similarly equipped with safety features

- a safe woodworking or craft shop, therapeutic and enjoyable, for residents who are accustomed to these activities
- a supportive social atmosphere and a daily routine that is tailored to the needs and abilities of the cognitively impaired
- a daily schedule of activities geared toward the residents' lifetime work and leisure experience and preferences, each modified to accommodate the residents' needs or limitations
- a host of activities that promote group interaction, discussion, and community that helps residents to exercise their social and communication skills

The hallmark of most new assisted-living facilities is their residential, homelike atmosphere and decor. An important component of the care of persons with dementia is making them feel comfortable and at ease. Most people feel more comfortable in a residential, nonhospital-like setting. A residential setting typically has carpeting throughout, living rooms and kitchens that look like those in someone's home, porches and gardens, and, often, private bedrooms.

The need for assistance with activities of daily living (ADLs) such as dressing, bathing, eating, and toileting, is a major reason for placement in an assisted-living facility. It is this critical element of service that varies most widely among assisted-living facilities.[7] The marketing information of many facilities promote the concept of "aging in place." "Aging in place" is the notion that even as a progressively disabling or terminal illness advances, a person can remain in an assisted-living facility (or one's own home) and be adequately cared for. The reality of "aging in place" can be much different than what is presented in a marketing brochure. Very few assisted-living facilities are staffed to provide for the highest physical and psychosocial functioning of an FTD patient who ages toward the final stages of life.

Once a person reaches a point where extensive or total care by staff is needed for certain ADLs, the amount of staff time needed just for that one resident increases significantly. The number of staff needed to provide extensive or total care with these ADLs, and the necessary skills training for this staff, are not things that can be taken for granted in the largely unregulated assisted-living setting.

Very few states have laws regulating assisted living or mandating minimum staffing or training levels. It is absolutely critical for those responsible for placing someone in an assisted-living facility to recognize signs of significant decline in functioning and to recognize the need for appropriate interventions. The responsible party must be vigilant in determining whether the assisted-living facility resident's needs are being met or whether another care setting is appropriate.

To determine if a person's needs are being adequately met in an assisted-living facility, the responsible party should use the same analysis described in the previous section on determining if nursing home placement is appropriate.

There are several characteristics of assisted-living facility staff that should be noted. While there is usually a nurse on staff, most of the care is provided by personal care attendants who are unlicensed and uncertified. The multitask worker is a hallmark of assisted-living care. A personal care attendant is usually a combination housekeeper, laundry aide, meal preparer, meal server, activities leader, and medication administrator, *as well as* the provider of ADL care (assistance with dressing, eating, toileting, incontinence care, bathing, etc.).[8] *One practice to be aware of that is widespread in the assisted-living setting is the administration of medications by unlicensed, nonnurse staff.* There are a number of drugs that are commonly used in the elderly and in people with dementia that require vigilant monitoring for negative side effects.

Other conditions or treatments that may require a greater level of expertise than might typically be found at an assisted-living facility are respiratory/oxygen treatments; wound care; colostomy/ostomy care; injections; catheterization; IV medications; tube feeding; and physical, occupational, or speech therapy. If a special therapeutic diet or special food consistency (e.g., pureed or mechanical soft food,* thickened liquids) is required, a dietician's input and oversight may be necessary.

It is important to know in advance if the facility charges additional fees when more assistance with ADL care is needed, particularly whether there is an additional charge for incontinence care. The cost for private-duty aides or nursing personnel is borne by the resident and is in addition to the basic monthly fee for the assisted-living facility.

When looking for a good assisted-living facility, some of the

---

*Mechanical soft foods are those that are "naturally" soft, like sloppy joes, tuna fish, or cottage cheese, or foods that are made soft, but not pureed, with a food processor.

resources identified in the previous section on finding a good nursing home apply as well. The local chapter of the Alzheimer's Association, especially participants in the chapter's caregiver support groups, can be very helpful. Also, the ombudsman in your county's Area Agency on Aging, the National Citizens Coalition for Nursing Home Reform,[9] and the Consumer Consortium on Assisted Living[10] can be good sources of information.

The suggestions in the previous section on what to look for and what and whom to ask during a visit to a nursing home should be followed precisely when visiting an assisted-living facility. The availability and acceptance of Medicaid or Supplemental Security Income (SSI) for coverage of assisted-living facility costs is extremely limited.[11]

Conclusion

For the most part, assisted living remains an option only for those who can afford it. A facility designed for people with dementia can be an ideal setting, providing a comfortable, noninstitutional environment where activities and routines are tailored to the abilities of the residents. Safety, monitoring, and assistance with medications and most activities of daily living can be provided in a familiar, supportive, residential atmosphere.

Because of the variation in the level of services provided by different assisted-living facilities, the responsible party must continually monitor for changes in condition that require additional assistance with care and the implementation of appropriate interventions. Continually look for specific signs of decline and determine whether the services provided by the facility have been increased to include the interventions needed to ensure the resident's highest level of physical and psychosocial functioning. If the resident's needs have increased but staff support and assistance has not, and/or avoidable conditions have developed, it is time to consider placement in another setting. If a resident's care needs are being met, an assisted-living facility can be much more comfortable and homelike than a nursing home.

NOTES

1. National Citizens Coalition for Nursing Home Reform, 1424 16th St., N.W., Ste. 202, Washington, DC 20036, 202-332-2275, www.nccnhr.org.

2. CMS, formerly the Health Care Financing Administration (HCFA), is the federal agency that oversees all nursing home care and Medicare and Medicaid funding. www.cms.hhs.gov.

3. Pennsylvania Department of Health, www.health.state.pa.us/qa/ltc.

4. Maryland Department of Health, www.mhcc.state.md.us.

5. Calculated by taking the number of nurses and nursing assistants working in a twenty-four-hour period, multiplying that total by the hours they each work (usually eight hours each), and dividing into that amount the number of residents in the facility in that twenty-four-hour period.

6. Generally, the first shift is 7:00 A.M.–3:00 P.M., second shift is 3:00 P.M.–11:00 P.M., third shift is 11:00 P.M.–7:00 A.M.

7. Catherine Hawes, Miriam Rose, and Charles D. Phillips, "A national study of assisted living for the frail elderly—Results of a national survey of facilities," Myers Research Institute (December 1999): 9–11, 17–18, and 54–62; Catherine Hawes and Charles D. Phillips, "High service or high privacy assisted living facilities, their residents and staff: Results from a national survey," U.S. Dept. of Health and Human Services, Texas A&M University, Miriam Rose, Myers Research Institute (November 2000):15–17.

8. Hawes and Phillips, "High service or high privacy assisted living," p. 41, 51, and 60.

9. See note 1.

10. Consumer Consortium on Assisted Living, 2342 Oak St., Falls Church, VA 22046, 703-533-8121, www.ccal.org.

11. Hawes and Phillips, "High service or high privacy assisted living," p. 56.

CHAPTER 20

By the Hands of Others:

Creating Helpful Support Networks

HELEN-ANN COMSTOCK

Responding to the challenge of caring for someone with frontotemporal dementia is never easy; it is demanding, frustrating, and stressful. Caregivers face the constant task of balancing the needs of the patient with their own needs and often those of other family members, as well. It's easy to feel overwhelmed. Caregiving requires a lot of individual effort, but it cannot be handled alone. Other people must be drawn in. By working together and sharing responsibilities, you and they can make life better for the person with frontotemporal dementia and for you, the caregiver. It is important, even lifesaving, to share the responsibility of caring and to develop your own support network. Having a support network has been shown to have "direct and stress-buffering effects"[1] on well-being. A support network allows you to provide needed assistance to the person with FTD while at the same time keeping a balance in other aspects of your life.

SETTING UP A SUPPORT NETWORK

The key to successfully coping with FTD is planning and establishing a support network. Here are the steps to follow.

1. *Educate yourself about the disease and its progression.* Knowledge of the disease will help you to understand how the disease affects your family member's behavior. It will help you to know what to expect over the course of the disease. Educating yourself about the disease is absolutely critical. A resource list for information specific to FTD is at the end of this chapter and at the end of this book. (See chapters 1 through 8 for more information.)

2. *Understand what is happening to your family member. This is the key to learning how to cope with the disease.* Think for a moment about the fact that your family member is losing his ability to cope with everyday living. He is losing his ability to be in control of his life. He still has wants and needs, but he is unable to express these desires or fulfill them himself. He is constantly failing to perform in a world where he used to be able to do everything. That's very scary! And people are individuals and react differently to this situation. Some become anxious and withdraw. Some express their frustration by striking out or running off. Some say impolite or even rude or crude things. Some exhibit inappropriate social or sexual behaviors. Family life is seriously disrupted by FTD. This is why it is so important to learn about the disease and ways to cope with it.

Caregivers who view a patient's memory and behavioral problems as a direct consequence of the disease generally are less bothered by them than caregivers who continue to view such problems as being in the patient's control. It's important to realize that the person with dementia is not in control of his behavior. It is the caregiver who is in control and who needs to change and adapt, because the person with dementia can't. Understanding the disease will aid you in making plans for care, and you will become a better caregiver.

3. *Tell your family and friends about the diagnosis and what it means.* Family and friends need to understand what is happening to your loved one if you are to have their support and help. Provide them with information about the disease: Give them a brochure or a fact sheet. This will help them to see why your loved one's behavior has changed. It will help them to realize that there is a neurological reason for the changes in behavior. They will learn that the changes are due to the disease and that your loved one has no control over the changes that are taking place, nor is she able to control her behavior.

Most people will find that what is happening to your family member is painful and frightening. Therefore, do not be hurt or surprised if they do not jump right in and offer to help. They need time to adjust to the situation. Give them time to learn and understand about the disease and, generally, they will overcome their fears and be supportive. However, be tolerant of those who are not able to overcome their discomfort and who may never be able to visit with your family member or assist with her care. They may offer to help in other ways that are useful to you, the caregiver, and thus become part of your support network.

4. *Ask for help.* It can't be stressed enough how very important it is to draw family members and friends into your support network. Don't be too proud or timid to ask for their help. Caring for someone with a frontotemporal dementia is never easy. You need all the help you can get! Not only will you, the caregiver, benefit from the support of family members and friends, your loved one will also, and so will your family.

In her helpful book, *Dear Aunt S: How to Ask for Help from Family and Friends in Time of Crisis,* Marion Cohen, Ph.D., writes, "Mostly I had to arrive at the mind-set that it was a crisis we were going through, that it was appropriate to ask for help, and that I had a right to do so—the right to gather a support system." She also points out that asking for help is a commitment toward fulfilling your responsibility toward the ill person, as he has a right to more people helping him.[2]

When you are planning to ask for help, be sure to think about all the people who might be able to provide various kinds of help. Include (1) people with whom you live; (2) family/relatives; (3) friends; (4) people from work or school; (5) people from clubs, organizations, or religious groups; (6) neighbors; and (7) agencies or other formal service providers. [3]

You can go about asking for help in different ways. In my situation, we were living in California when my husband was diagnosed with FTD and all our family were living on the East Coast, so I needed to depend on friends for help. I had a wine and cheese party and invited all our friends. During the party I spoke briefly about my husband's diagnosis and gave out an information sheet. I said that even though my husband was losing his ability to do many things, he still needed companionship and stimulation, and I needed a break from twenty-four-hour-a-day caregiving. I asked them to help on a regular basis (it's important to have a regular commitment) in any way they could, such as taking my husband for walks, playing card games, doing puzzles, and working on reading skills or math problems (he was a math professor). At the end of the evening, twenty-five people (working professionals as well as community volunteers) each committed to spend one hour a week with my husband. One friend even came up with her own idea to help: She saved her errands and took my husband along in her car once a week while she did her errands. He loved the ride in the car and her company, even though he was unable to converse.

This support network helped us in so many ways. It kept us from the isolation that so many families experience when coping with FTD. It provided my husband with companionship. It gave me some breaks, which allowed me to go to the grocery store, take a walk on my own, visit a friend, etc. And, since our volunteers mostly were parents of our children's friends, it helped their children to have a better understanding of what was happening to our family. Of course, as the disease progressed and my husband lost his ability to speak and his attention span dropped to less than five minutes, changes needed to be made in the program. By that time, walks, rides in the car, and simple games were the most useful. Daycare became a helpful option. It was a place where my husband could be part of the activities, even though he could not participate in them, and a service that gave me some respite.

Now, you may not be comfortable with having a wine and cheese party or some other sort of gathering to set up your support network. In her book, Dr. Cohen outlines another way to set up a support network. She suggests the following: Write "asking-for-help" letters, and she gives very detailed suggestions about how to do this, as well as how to arrange a family meeting. Writing letters (or e-mails, if you prefer) allows you to tell about your situation without interruption, and it allows the recipient the time and space to reflect and to get used to the idea. You can offer specific suggestions for how the recipient can help: Visit with your family member, drive him to day care, help with finding resources, invite the caregiver for something fun, include both caregiver and patient in informal gatherings, etc. Use your creativity; the list of options will vary with each family situation.

In asking for help, try to find a good friend or family member who will take on the asking role for you—someone to act as your advocate. People will be more comfortable talking with a third party. They'll feel more free to ask questions and reveal their fears and discomfort about helping. Your advocate can be invaluable.

5. *Join a support group.* A support group is another important piece of your support network. Joining a support group gives you the opportunity to meet other people who are experiencing the same problems and griefs as you are. They also provide information about FTD and local resources. There is much you can learn from the experience of other members and their sympathetic understanding of your situation. Support groups specific to FTD are the most helpful, but they are available only in limited areas. Contact the Association for Frontotemporal Dementias for the location of FTD-specific support groups, or check with your local Alzheimer's Association chapter or local medical center to see if they have an FTD-specific support group.

If you are unable to locate an FTD-specific support group, try an Alzheimer's support group. You still will learn about local resources and find companionship from group members.

If you are unable to leave your family member to attend a support group meeting or if there is no nearby support group, ask if there is a telephone support group or an on-line support group. Or, ask if you can be linked up to another caregiver who will become your telephone buddy. I found such an arrangement extremely helpful when I was unable to leave my husband to attend a support group. Being a telephone buddy is a two-way arrangement. Telephone buddies offer each other support and helpful suggestions during difficult times, but they also share amusing incidents or poignant moments. Having a telephone buddy is the next best thing to having a sympathetic friend stop by for a cup of coffee or a glass of wine.

6. *Make use of respite resources.* Adult daycare provides benefits to the person with FTD and eases the caregiving burden. It allows the caregiver time to return to work or take care of personal needs. It gives the person with FTD an opportunity for socialization and stimulation. In-home or overnight institutional respite gives the caregiver and/or family an opportunity for much-needed relief.

7. *Take care of yourself.* Caregiver members of the FTD Support Group of the Orange County (CA) Chapter of the Alzheimer's Association were asked to answer the question, "What's the most important piece of advice you would give to someone who has just become a caregiver for a person with FTD?" Overwhelmingly, their response was: *"The first thing to do is take care of yourself."* Here's what they suggest to accomplish this: Keep up spiritual, social, and community activities; exercise; be open to talking with a therapist knowledgeable about FTD; give yourself permission to be "selfish." And learn, learn, learn! Learn to be patient; learn that your relationship with the family member with FTD will change; learn to lower your expectations of what the person with FTD can do (but always keep in mind that she is an adult, not a child), learn about the disease; learn to accept help; learn that it is all right and healthy to laugh. Keep your sense of humor!

To this excellent advice from experienced caregivers, I would add, learn to remember love. The person with FTD may not remember much. Eventually she may not seem to know you or respond to anything. She may not show pain or fear or loneliness, but I believe she experiences them. She may not remember your gentle touch, kind words or hugs, but I believe she feels them. She may no longer be able to do anything. But I believe she still remembers love and feels your loving care.

Follow the seven steps to set up a support network for yourself so that you will be able to give that loving care.

RESOURCES

Medical Centers and Organizations

Medical Centers. If you obtained the diagnosis at a university medical center, you should be able to obtain information from the center. Some centers also offer family consultations and maintain support groups.

The Association for Frontotemporal Dementias (AFTD), P.O. Box 7191, St. David's, PA 19087-7191. A new nationwide nonprofit organization whose mission is to promote and fund research into finding the cause and cure for frontotemporal dementias; to

provide information, education, and support to persons diagnosed with FTD and their families and caregivers; and to educate physicians and allied health professionals about FTD.
www.FTD-Picks.org.

Alzheimer's Association (USA), 919 N. Michigan Ave., Ste. 1100,
Chicago, IL 60611-1676. (800-272-3900 national Helpline),
www.alz.org. The association publishes a variety of useful
brochures (ask for "Related Disorders," among others). The
Summer 2001 issue of the Association's *Advances* has an article
on frontotemporal dementia. See www.alz.org/caregiver/pro-
grams/advances.

Association chapters maintain local support groups, lists of daycare
centers, in-home care providers, nursing homes, and information
about drugs, clinical trials, research, and care tips. Many association
chapters also offer family caregiver training, and this is most valuable as you cope with caring for your family member. I especially
urge you to arrange to participate in caregiver training, although it
is geared toward Alzheimer's, because much of the information and
many of the care tips are helpful for FTD as well.

In addition to the United States Alzheimer's Association and its
many chapters, excellent information is available from international
Alzheimer's associations or societies.

Alzheimer's Society, United Kingdom, Gordon House, 10 Greencoat
Pl., London SW1P 1PH UK. Information Sheet, "What is frontotemporal dementia (including Pick's disease)?" www.
alzheimers.org.uk.

Alzheimer's Australia, P. O. Box 108, Higgins, ACT 2615, Australia.
Excellent Help Notes specific to Pick's and frontal lobe
dementia, reading list. www.alzheimers.org.au.

Society for Progressive Supranuclear Palsy, Woodholme Medical Bldg.,
Ste. 515, 1828 GreeneTree Rd., Baltimore, MD 21208 (U.S. 410-
486-3330; 800-457-4777) (Canada toll-free 866-457-4777). The
society promotes and funds research into finding the cause and
cure for progressive supranuclear palsy (PSP). It provides information, education, support, and advocacy to persons diagnosed
with PSP, their families, and caregivers. The society also edu-

cates physicians and allied health professionals on PSP and how to improve patient care. www.psp.org.

ADEAR (Alzheimer's Disease Education and Research), National Institute on Aging, P.O. Box 8250, Silver Spring, MD 20907-8250, (800-438-4380). The publication, *Connections,* March 2002 issue, volume 9, no. 4, focuses on frontotemporal dementia. It has the most comprehensive information available at the time of this book's printing. www.alzheimers.org/pubs/conv099n4.html.

NINDS (National Institute of Neurological Disorders and Stroke), National Institutes of Health, 31 Center Dr., Bethesda, MD 20892. Fact sheets on Pick's disease, dementia with Lewy bodies, progressive supranuclear palsy, and corticobasal degeneration. www.ninds.nih.gov.

Dementia Research Group, United Kingdom, The National Hospital for Neurology and Neurosurgery, Queen Square, London WC1N 3BG, UK. www.dementia.ion.ucl.ac.uk. Click on CANDID (Counseling ANd Diagnosis In Dementia) for a wealth of information specific to FTD: Pick's disease support group, fact sheets, articles, books, newsletter. Or go directly to CANDID, www.pdsg.uk.

Family Caregiver Alliance, 690 Market St., Ste. 600, San Francisco, CA 94104 (415-434-3388). Founded in 1977, the first community-based nonprofit organization in the U.S. to address the needs of families and friends providing long-term care at home. Fact sheets on various dementias, as well as caregiver issues, statistics, and demographics. www.caregiver.org/factsheets. Interview with Dr. Bruce Miller, UCSF, www.caregiver.org/interviews/bmiller/html.

National Organization for Rare Disorders, Inc. (NORD), P.O. Box 8923, New Fairfield, CT 06812-8923 (203-746-6518) www.rarediseases.org. Search "Rare Diseases Database—Alphabetical Listing," scroll down to Corticobasal, Pick's disease, etc., for brief information about the disease and information about organizations offering help. There is a small charge for full-text reports.

Eldercare Locator

This is a nationwide, toll-free service that helps older adults and their caregivers find local services for seniors. Eldercare Locator links to information and referral services of each state and to area agencies on aging. 800-677-1116 or www.eldercare.gov.

Area Agencies on Aging (U.S.)

These agencies provide many helpful long-term care services to patients and families. You may apply for state and federal financial aid (Medicaid) for home care and nursing home care through your local Area Agency on Aging. Listings for Area Agencies on Aging are located under "Guide to Human Services" in the blue pages of the telephone directory.

Web Sites (in addition to those previously noted)

PubMed, a service of the National Library of Medicine, National Institutes of Health, provides access to MEDLINE citations and includes links to many sites providing full-text articles and other related resources, at www.ncbi.nlm.nih.gov. Click on PubMed; search on PubMed for Pick's disease, frontotemporal dementia, Lewy body, etc.

Emedicine, "Pick's Disease," authored by Anna M. Barrett, M.D., Pennsylvania State University, College of Medicine, from *eMedicine Journal*, Nov. 27, 2001, vol. 2, no. 11. www.emedicine.com.

Articles

Many excellent articles are in print, and many can be found on-line by typing "Pick's disease" or "frontotemporal dementia." The following are particularly useful.

Chow, Tiffany. "How to recognize frontotemporal dementia." *Neuropsychiatry Reviews* 3, no. 3 (April 2002). Tiffany Chow, M.D., a member of the Work Group on Frontotemporal Dementia and Pick's Disease, describes key manifestations of FTD and suggests tips that can aid diagnosis. She also offers advice on how to treat the behavioral and cognitive components of FTD. [Online], www.neuropsychiatryreviews.com/apr02/recognize.html.

Grossman, Murray. "A Multidisciplinary approach to Pick's disease and frontotemporal dementia." *Neurology* 56, no. 11, suppl. 4 (2001).

McKhann, Guy M., et al. "Clinical and pathological diagnosis of frontotemporal dementia: Report of the work group on frontotemporal dementia and Pick's disease." *Archives of Neurology* 58, no. 11 (Nov. 2001).

Snowden, Julie S., David Neary, and David M. A. Mann. "Frontotemporal dementia." *British Journal of Psychiatry* 180 (2002). An overview of clinical and pathological characteristics of frontotemporal dementia and its nosological status. [Online], www.psychiatry.wustl.edu/Resources/LiteratureList/2002/February/Snowden.pdf.

Yeaworth, Rosalee C. "Use of the Internet in survey research." *Journal of Professional Nursing* 17, no. 4 (July–Aug. 2001). This survey of the Pick's Disease Network gathers data on patient and family experiences and other caregiver-related information.

Books

Erb, Clinton A. *Losing Lou-Ann*. Brandon, Vt.: Holistic Education Press, 1996. An inspiring account of a spouse caring for his wife with Pick's disease.

Kertesz, Andrew, and David G. Munoz. *Pick's Disease and Pick Complex*. Chichester, U.K.: Wiley-Liss, 1998. The first book devoted to Pick's disease and its clinical and pathological manifestations. A comprehensive reference that clarifies Pick's diagnosis compared to other forms of dementia.

NOTES

1. Elizabeth M. Tracy and James K. Whittaker, "The social network map: Assessing social support in clinical practice, families in society," *Journal of Contemporary Human Services* (1990).

2. Marion Cohen, Ph.D., *Dear Aunt S: How to Ask for Help from Family and Friends in Time of Crisis* (Brooklyn, N.Y.: Center for Thanatology Research, 2003).

3. Tracy and Whittaker, "The social network map."

CHAPTER 21

Money Matters:

Securing Financial and Legal Readiness

PAUL L. FELDMAN AND KENT S. JAMISON

INTRODUCTION

Planning for the financial and legal consequences of a family member with FTD is a formidable challenge because of the many complex and difficult issues that must be addressed. The issues range from legal matters when your family member becomes unable to make those types of decisions for themselves, to financial considerations over how the cost of care (either at home or in an institutionalized setting) will be met. Financial issues involve strategies for taking full advantage of all insurance- and government-funded programs for the direct cost of care. Also, indirect issues include ways of replacing lost income, maximizing tax deductions, and developing strategies for preserving assets for the future needs of any remaining family members.

Since FTD is a progressive, degenerative disease that leads to gradual loss of decision-making functioning, these issues intensify as the level of function of the individual declines. The difficulty of developing a plan can vary tremendously depending on course of the illness and the particular strengths and adaptability of the social and family network the caregiver has to draw upon. Moreover, the steps taken can also be dictated by whether the family member with FTD is married or single, and if the principal caregiver is an adult child or some other relative. Since FTD often strikes at relatively young ages, the financial strategies for meeting the costs of care can also differ depending on whether or not the person (and the spouse, if married) is under the age of sixty-five, or in some instances, under the age of sixty.

This chapter will attempt to lay out the principal legal and financial issues that must be faced in caring for someone with FTD. The goal of this chapter is to provide strategies for seeking out resources to help develop a customized care plan that works for you and your family. It will identify core programs that will be helpful and pinpoint some of the obstacles that you may have to overcome due to the uniqueness of FTD when applying for these programs. A thorough review of this chapter should establish a solid foundation upon which you can then seek the individualized advice you will need.

No one person can provide all the information you will need to make these decisions. One reality of our healthcare system is that there is no case manager. Each caregiver must put together what is best for him and his loved one depending on his own needs, and what he and his loved one may qualify for. Caregivers should be aware that estate lawyers and certified financial planners, while competent within their own spheres of expertise, may not be adequately versed in the complexities you are likely to be faced with in this situation. Some of the best professionals available practice in the area now known as Elder Law. One should be particularly cautious about information picked up from other caregivers or lay people. While these can be useful starting points, caregivers and other family members must be careful not to be lulled into believing that the financial information being volunteered is the best or only option. Many individualized factors that are particular to one situation may be inappropriate for your circumstances. Caregivers need to be mindful that these are areas where small differences can dictate large differences in how one plans for these eventualities.

GENERAL RESOURCES

A good first step should be to contact your local Alzheimer's Association chapter. Be aware that there are vast differences in the size and sophistication of local chapters. While the official name of the organization is the Alzheimer's Disease and Related Disorders Association, the reality is that only a handful of chapters have much specific information pertaining to FTD. Nonetheless, many of the programs and legal steps that are needed for FTD are the same as for Alzheimer's and so this can still be an important first step. If your local chapter does not have what you need, don't hesitate to contact a larger chapter in a more urbanized area. Since many programs are state specific, your first priority should be to contact other chapters within your state, then larger chapters in other states. If you don't find what you're looking for through the Alzheimer's Association, consider branching out by calling or reviewing the web sites of chapters of other neurological degenerative diseases such as Parkinson's or multiple sclerosis. While these diseases may be different, many of the caregiving issues are similar enough to be useful. There are also various caregiver associations such as the Family Caregiver Alliance, the Well Spouse Foundation, or the National Family Caregivers Association.

SURROGATE DECISION MAKING

Unlike other illnesses, all dementias, not just FTD, render the individual incapable of handling their own affairs. These may be financial or legal in nature and can range from something as simple as endorsing a check to something as serious as end-of-life issues. There are a number of legal instruments designed to cover these contingencies, the most common of which is a durable power of attorney, but healthcare directives and a living will can also be employed. These instruments transfer to someone else the legal authority for acting in the best interest of the person while she is still alive. A will and a trust are legal instruments for passing property to others after the person dies, though trusts can sometimes be used to provide for the person financially while she is still alive. All of these legal instruments are largely governed by state law and should be executed in the state in which you reside. It is strongly suggested that you seek an attorney licensed in your state who regularly practices in Elder Law. If any of these documents are already in place, an attorney in the state in which you are now residing should review them. They should review that the documents are compatible with current state laws and applicable to your current situation. Because of the degenerative nature of FTD, it is important that these legal documents get put into place as soon as possible.

VOLUNTARY ARRANGEMENTS

Durable Power of Attorney

The most common voluntary arrangement that an individual with FTD establishes is one controlled by a durable power of attorney (POA), either for financial purposes and/or for medical purposes (including end-of-life care decision making). The document designates someone else (or several individuals) to be the agent to make decisions in the specific areas authorized by the document. A properly drawn document that designates only one agent should have a successor designated if the primary individual cannot provide the appropriate assistance.

The document should list certain authority for the agent to make decisions. The authority given would be for such things as selling or transferring real estate, banking decisions, entering a safe deposit box, filing tax returns, the ability to handle pension and Social Security as well as any other area for which the individual can no longer make decisions. Especially important is the ability to undertake financial planning to deal with the issues involved with government entitlements, principally Medicaid.

It is helpful to have several (at least four) original copies of this document executed since someone being asked to rely upon this document (such as a title company involved in a real estate transaction) will often wish to retain an original. It is also helpful when executing a general POA that you obtain forms from the bank at which your family member's primary checking account is located. Once the forms from the financial institution are obtained and executed, it is sometimes easier to have one's authority under a POA already registered.

There is a difference between being listed on a bank account as a power of attorney, which means that you have the ability to access the account, and being listed as a joint owner. A joint owner also has the ability to access the account, but at the death of one of the joint owners, the account is owned by the surviving joint owner and is not controlled by the will of the deceased individual with FTD. There is a tax benefit to having it owned jointly if your family member with FTD predeceases you. In the unlikely event that you predecease your family member and the account was jointly owned, your family member might be taxed on his or her own money. In the case of a spouse, most joint accounts should be changed to the name of the well-spouse alone, or well-spouse with another family member such as an adult child.

Handling of a Social Security check can be done without a power of attorney by utilizing the procedure established by the Social Security Administration to become the representative payee. This is exclusively a federal program administered under extensive federal regulations. An individual can authorize someone to be the representative payee to receive that individual's check to be deposited into an account in the name of the representative payee and administered for the benefit of the recipient. The regulations also provide that if the individual cannot voluntarily authorize someone to be the representative payee, after a physician certifies that the recipient is unable to handle his own check, Social Security can designate an individual from a prioritized list of those who are eligible. This can be done by direct deposit (checks can even be directly deposited to a nursing home).

A general POA can provide your agent the authority to make medical care decisions, or withhold authorizing certain medical care decisions (or withdrawing consent after having previously authorized a medical decision). You can separate the authority to make medical care decisions from the authority to make financial decisions, similar to separating the guardianship of a person from the guardianship of an estate.

Living Will

If you have a Medical POA, it can also provide for end-of-life care decisions in the nature of a "living will" (legally known as an advance directive). One can have a living will and a medical power of attorney (with different decision makers). The most important aspect is making sure that the healthcare provider knows of the existence of this document. This document will express the intentions of your family member at a time when he or she cannot express them herself.

As the family member declines, these documents should be conveniently located so they can be retrieved on short notice. Caregivers need to be aware that ambulance crews, as paraprofessionals, cannot legally follow healthcare directives because they are not under the direct supervision of a physician until they reach the hospital. Even emergency rooms may be reluctant to follow the directives. Caregivers need to assert themselves if faced with this by presenting a copy of the directives and insisting the instructions be followed.

Trusts

Another voluntary arrangement to handle just the financial affairs of an individual with FTD is the establishment of a trust. A trust is a legal arrangement between individuals. The one who sets it up (usually done by the impaired individual or a family member under a POA) is known as the settlor or grantor. The person managing the fund is known as the trustee, and the person who benefits from the trust is known as the lifetime beneficiary. Upon the death of the lifetime beneficiary, the trust acts as a will and passes whatever assets remain in the trust to the designated remainder beneficiaries. A trust is generally used only when there are significant assets or special circumstances, such as the financial support of more than one person, which would justify the expense incurred in administering a trust, including the bookkeeping and/or the extra tax returns that would have to be prepared.

In the case of a spouse, a preexisting will needs to be updated so that, in the unlikely event the well-spouse dies, their estate will not transfer to the impaired spouse with FTD. In this circumstance, setting up an unfunded trust is ideal. In an unfunded living trust, no assets need be transferred. Only upon death (or disability, if so specified in the trust document) would assets be transferred. The trust can be drawn up to specify how the assets would be used to care for the impaired spouse with FTD.

In rare instances, when the individual suffering from FTD either refuses to plan or has reached a point where she is unable to plan, the family or caregiver may be left with no alternative but to go to court to declare the person incompetent. The steps involved in this are covered in the next section.

INVOLUNTARY ARRANGEMENTS

One of the major challenges of FTD is that a person can be very high functioning in some areas while experiencing severe deficits in others. This can occur in the early stages of the disease. Such a person may be able to function but without appropriate judgment. In this case, the caregiver may establish a guardianship or conservatorship in a court proceeding. A guardianship is established by going to a lawyer to prepare a petition or complaint to be filed in the trial division of your state court system (sometimes known as the orphans' court or surrogate court, depending on the state) and having a hearing in front of a judge. Medical testimony is presented and, depending upon the specific jurisdiction, the alleged incapacitated person may or may not be required to attend the hearing. Also depending upon the jurisdiction, an attorney for the alleged incapacitated person, separate from the individual who is petitioning the court, sometimes must be appointed.

If the judge decides that the individual is unable to receive and evaluate information effectively and make appropriate decisions based upon that information, that judge may appoint either a limited or a plenary guardian to be responsible for financial and/or personal decisions. If you were to file for a guardian, for example, to be appointed to handle only the finances at a time when your family member can still make medical decisions, you might be required to file again later to have a guardian appointed for making medical decisions when the disease progresses further. Even if the individual is relatively high functioning and able to express his opposition to being defined as incapacitated, the judge can find that the individual's executive functioning (i.e., decision making) is impaired to such an extent that a guardian is warranted. The court will then have supervision over the financial decisions that must be made.

All of the voluntary or involuntary arrangements established to address this issue have advantages and disadvantages to each of them. If pursuing a guardianship becomes necessary, one should have a clear understanding of the restrictions and procedures before proceeding to establish one.

The guardianship provisions are usually separate and distinct from regulations when a commitment, either involuntary or voluntary, is needed under a state's Mental Health Act. If an individual is so impaired and his actions are so likely to pose an immediate risk of harm, either to himself or to others, a person could be temporarily admitted to a psychiatric care facility to prevent harm. Since this can be an immediate detainment by the local health department, an individual must be given a hearing within a very short time after the commitment (usually three to five days). These involuntary commitments under the Mental Health Act can be extended for short periods of time and also converted to a voluntary commitment, should the individual understand the immediate need for care. A commitment under the Mental Health Act is not an alternative to proceeding under the guardianship provisions of state law, since the goal of the former is treatment and the goal of the latter is decision making.

ISSUES AFFECTING INCOME

Income Related

An individual with FTD eventually will become incapacitated and unable to work. If the individual has already retired, he may be receiving Old Age Retirement Benefits under the Social Security Act, which would not be effected by his incapacity. However, one must be a certain age (currently sixty-five) to receive normal benefits. One can retire sooner, as early as sixty-two, but at reduced benefits. If one is sixty-five or older and receiving Social Security, she is already eligible for Medicare.

If a person is younger than sixty-five and has generally worked twenty quarters (five years) in the past ten years prior to the onset of the disability, the individual will be eligible for Social Security Disability. Two years after qualifying for disability, an individual is entitled to Medicare. Federal law governs all these programs. The programs are not dependent upon one's other resources (such as the well-spouse's income or pension). The amount received depends solely on the amount earned in previous years and the presence of any dependent children under the age of sixteen. The extra allocation for dependent children stops as each child turns sixteen.

To qualify, you must provide documentation of the diagnosis and that the person is terminally ill, and not mentally capable of applying for themselves. Your loved one need not be present when you apply but you do have to go in person to a local Social Security office. Social Security intake workers will help you. They will go back retroactively to when the disease first affected your loved one's employment status (which shortens the twenty-four-month wait for when the person becomes eligible for Medicare). Sometimes examinations by Social Security's own designated physician is required, but this is usually waived in the case of Alzheimer's and FTD. To find out more, contact your local Social Security office or check the Web at www.ssa.gov.

If an individual must leave work because of his incapacity, he is likely to be eligible for any disability coverage his employer may have. This coverage sometimes contains a Social Security offset clause limiting the total combined benefits from the employer's coverage and Social Security to no more than 70 percent of the employee's former income. Your family member may own an individual disability income policy of his own. This is most often the case for certain professionals and self-employed individuals. Contact the agent representing the insurer to see about filing a claim. Some disability income policies are written in such a way that they cover you if you cannot perform the duties of your "own occupation." Others are more restrictive and only provide coverage if you cannot work at all. Obviously, which type it is can affect how soon your loved one will be declared eligible.

If an individual is unable to work and is disabled but does not have a sufficient work record to qualify for Social Security Disability, then that person can qualify for Supplemental Security Income, which provides income up to minimum poverty levels, which is approximately $550.00 a month. If that is the case, an individual will also qualify for Medical Assistance (Medicaid), which is a federal program administered by individual states.

One source that may be able to be tapped for income is an IRA. The normal penalty for early withdrawals imposed on those under the age of fifty-nine is waived if the person is disabled.

Expense Related—Deductibility

There are some income tax consequences about which an individual should be aware. It is likely that one will incur expenses for nursing home care, personal care in a facility, or companion care at home (depending upon the level of functioning that the individual with FTD is able to achieve). These are considered to be medical expenses, which are deductible for income tax purposes to the extent that they exceed 7.5 percent (2002) of your adjusted gross income. Having a good accountant to do this end-of-the-year planning will pay for itself.

Expense Related—Dependent Care Allowance

This program is most often used as a tax credit for parents with children in some type of child care arrangement, but it can also be used by any wage earner caring for a disabled family member. Under the provisions of the dependent care allowance, you are allowed to set aside up to $5,000 if married, or $2,500 if single, of earned income to pay for the costs in caring for a disabled dependent living in your home. The money set aside is not subject to federal income tax and possibly state income tax, depending on the state in which you reside. (Note that the money spent on care from the amount set aside can still go toward satisfying the 7.5 percent medical expense deductible.)

COVERING THE COST OF MEDICAL CARE

It is difficult to provide a blanket description of how the expenses of caring for your loved one at home will be covered. It can depend so much on the particular type of expenditure, the provisions of your health plan, and unfortunately, all too often, technicalities. The problem is that the type of treatment most often called for to care for someone with dementia does not fit the traditional "medical model" for which these plans were designed. The fact it is FTD often only compounds the problem further. For most people, it is a question of what will be covered and how well. The two main coverage sources for those under sixty-five are private health insurance (primarily through an employer) and eventually Medicare (once the twenty-four-month waiting period after qualifying for Social Security Disability ends). For those already sixty-five or over, it most likely will be Medicare and Medigap. Someone without enough prior work experience to qualify for Social Security Disability may qualify for Supplemental Security Disability Income (SSDI), depending on asset and income limitations. If qualified, then she will then also qualify for Medicaid, a comprehensive healthcare program for those with low income.

For Those under Sixty-five

The main coverage will be group health insurance, either through the employer of the individual with FTD or the spouse's employer. If it is the former, coverage *may* continue if the individual qualifies for disability income through that employer. If not, coverage will continue after the person leaves employment for up to twenty-four months under COBRA. However, while COBRA assures that coverage continues, the family must pay the full premium (i.e., the employer's share as well as the employee's). This can be a substantial amount (these premiums can, however, be counted as a deductible medical expense as explained earlier.) When COBRA coverage ceases after twenty-four months, the person (and any children under the age of sixteen) will be covered under Medicare if they qualified for Social Security Disability twenty-four months earlier.

Unless the spouse has coverage through his or her own place of employment, the well-spouse may be left without coverage. There are no good solutions to this. A spouse in this situation should check into the professional associations they belong to or could join. If either person is fifty or over, they can join AARP.

In terms of the types of expenses, doctor's visits, lab tests, and prescriptions are usually covered under private health insurance. A professional therapist for the person with FTD is probably covered (a psychiatrist is likely to be called upon to prescribe medications that will help control the behaviors of the person in his dementia). Hospitalization is likely to be covered. However, the type of hospitalization a person with FTD is most likely to need will be in an inpatient psychiatric facility, and that may or may not be covered. If it is covered, there are stricter limitations than for a regular hospitalization. What is not likely to be covered is the use of an adult day-care facility and a home health aide. Medicare only covers a home health aide if skilled care or physical, occupational, or speech therapy is also required. Skilled care means a nurse needs to perform medical procedures like dress a wound or change a catheter. Medicare also does not cover prescription drugs.

For Those Sixty-five and Over

The principal sources of coverage are likely to be Medicare and Medigap. Again, doctor's visits, lab work, and hospitalization (with restrictions on psychiatric admissions) will be covered. Home healthcare and adult care typically will not (unless as noted above for skilled care or physical, occupational, or speech therapy), nor will prescriptions. Important exceptions to this are waiver programs and the Medicare Life Care Program.

Exceptions under Medicare That Provide Broader Coverage

Under its Life Care Program, Medicare will underwrite the cost of adult daycare programs, *if* there is a skilled component. Such programs have a very large component of skilled care, such as counseling and other therapy, which is provided for individuals with FTD and enables them to remain at home longer. This program recognizes that keeping an individual healthy and at home is often not only less expensive but often a better option than placing her somewhere without the benefit of appropriate care suited to her dementia program. Also, some states have what is known as a waiver program to permit Medicaid to underwrite the cost of care at home, provided the other criteria necessary to establish eligibility have been met. Although this program does not provide twenty-four-hour care, it can provide up to approximately eight hours of care. Combining that with an adult daycare program might allow the impaired individual to be managed at home longer. However, since at times there are waiting lists of individuals who wish to enroll for this program, one should plan to apply for the waiver program at least six months to one year ahead of the time that you anticipate you will need it.

Other Sources of Coverage

There are at least two possible sources of coverage beyond private health insurance, Medicare, and Medicaid. One is long-term care policies. These policies for long-term care have begun to be more widely sold in the last five years. Many of these policies expressly provide for dementia. If the family member with FTD is fortunate enough to be covered under such a policy, he may also be covered for home healthcare, e.g., adult daycare and a home health aide (without needing skilled care). There may also be some limited state-funded programs. Your local Alzheimer's chapter may be your best source for finding out about these state specific programs.

CAREGIVER-RELATED ISSUES

Caring for a person with FTD can be very taxing and time consuming. Some caregivers try to hold down a job and take care of their loved one at the same time. There are two options caregivers can turn to for some relief.

Family Care Leave

Family members who are working for public agencies or private sector employers with fifty or more employees are eligible for leave under the Family Medical Leave Act (FMLA). To be eligible you must have worked for your employer for at least twelve months and have worked one thousand hours in the previous six months. You must be related to the family member with FTD but cannot be an "in-law." You do not have to be living with the FTD sufferer. You are allowed up to twelve weeks off work without pay. You are guaranteed your job or one equivalent when you return. You keep your benefits, but for employer-provided health insurance you must continue to pay the employee share. *You do not have to take all twelve weeks at once.* You must work this out with your employer. Employers require thirty days notice. Some states have their own family care leave programs that may be more generous than the federal program.

Respite Care

Sometimes caregivers need a break. Either they are exhausted or they have needs of their own that must be met. To deal with this difficult circumstance, they can turn to respite care. Respite care is placing the patient with FTD in a nursing home or similar overnight-supervised setting for a limited period, typically a few days or a week or two. Normally, this is not covered by any insurance because it is not medically necessary. However, some long-term care policies do provide for this and a few states have state-funded programs to help defray the costs. Your local Alzheimer's Association chapter can tell you whether there are any such programs in your state.

COVERING THE COST OF INSTITUTIONAL CARE

Medicare does *not* cover nursing home care except under limited circumstances, nor do most private health insurance plans. If the family has purchased a separate long-term care policy before the onset of the illness, some coverage will be possible. Even then, unless the most generous options were selected, the policy may not be enough to cover an extended long-term stay. What do families do? The answer is that the government steps in through Medicaid. Medicaid is a federal and state-funded program that covers nursing home costs for those without the means to pay.

When Medicare Does Pay

Two conditions must be met before Medicare will pay for nursing home care. First, the level of care required must be skilled nursing care, or physical or speech therapy. Second, the family member must have been hospitalized for at least three days prior to being discharged to a nursing home. Even under these limited circumstances, Medicare (along with most Medigap policies) will still only pay for up to one hundred days of care. In other words, Medicare is set up to facilitate recovery following a hospitalization and not for the kind of long-term institutionalization someone with dementia typically requires. Please note that this program will only pay for care in a certified facility.

Medicaid Eligibility

There are at least four levels of progressively intensive types of institutionalized care: *assisted living, custodial care, intermediate care,* and *skilled care.* As previously stated, Medicare will only pay for skilled nursing-home care and then only under certain circumstances. Medicaid does not require prior hospitalization, but still only covers intermediate or skilled care. The regulations governing the financial requirements for eligibility for Medicaid are very strict. While this is a federal program (with matching funds from the state) many of the limits governing eligibility are set by each state. Therefore, it is important to work with an Elder Care attorney or some other expert who is knowledgeable about the limits in your state. It is also important that this be done as far in advance as possible to maximize the funds the family has available and to provide the kind of detailed documentation of the family's finances the application process will later require.

To qualify for Medicaid, the program looks at the person's income and assets. If the person's income is less than the cost of the nursing home and the person has insufficient "available" assets to cover the cost of care, then Medicaid will pay. How the program looks at those assets and income depends on whether the person is married or not.

A single institutionalized individual is entitled to keep a minimum of assets for his or her spending needs, which is approximately $2,000 or $2,400 (the amount can vary between or even within a state depending on technicalities, plus the levels themselves can vary between states). Someone with more than allowed assets will have to "spend down" their funds to reach this level before Medicaid will begin paying. In addition, any income they have, such as Social Security or a pension, will go toward offsetting the amount Medicaid must pay—less $30 per month (or $35, again depending on the state), which is set aside for personal, nonmedical expenses such as a haircut or clothes.

There are some key assets that are exempt and not counted as part of the minimum assets to be retained for the individual. Medicaid allows the family member to set aside up to approximately $7,500 in prepaid funeral expenses (again, these levels can be set differently in different states). You can establish "an irrevocable burial reserve" by going to a funeral director directly and prepaying for the arrangements, or you can establish a restricted account at your local bank. Although you would not be able to access this $7,500, neither would you be required to spend these monies on your family member's medical care.

If the family member is married, a different set of rules govern assets and income. These rules are intended to leave the "community spouse" with enough money to meet his or her expenses. The community spouse is entitled to keep as much income as he or she earns. Also, the community spouse is entitled to an additional amount of the institutionalized spouse's income, if the community spouse's income is below a specified minimum amount (approximately $1,493 per month plus the shelter costs of the spouse living in the community in excess of $448 per month). Whatever income the community spouse cannot retain will all go to the nursing home except for $30 (or $35) a month.

The community spouse is also entitled to keep assets up to $89,300 (not counting the house, a car, and certain other exempt assets explained later). If the combined assets of both spouses (regardless of whose name these assets are in) exceeds $89,300 (the amount is adjusted each year for inflation) they must "spend down" to the $89,300 level before Medicaid will begin paying nursing home charges.

If the couple's combined assets exceed $89,300 there are several alternatives to spending the excess that will help preserve the family's assets. It is legitimate to spend excess assets on (1) paying down the mortgage since the house is excluded, (2) a home improvement because the house is excluded, or (3) a car. There is a penalty if money is transferred to someone else (e.g., another family member). What Medicaid does is delay the date they will begin paying nursing home costs measured by the amount transferred (the disqualified period). The penalty is dollar-for-dollar of nursing home costs for each dollar transferred. For example, if a couple has $20,000 in excess of $89,300, they could transfer $10,000 to another family member and then pay $10,000 in nursing home costs before they would qualify for Medicaid. (Warning: The amount of charges Medicaid will allow is set by Medicaid and is likely to be lower than the actual nursing home charges. For example, the nursing home may charge $150 a day but Medicaid will only allow $125. You will have to pay the difference as well. What this means is that you could end up paying more than $10,000 to offset the $10,000 gifted to someone else.) Whatever steps are taken will have to be documented when the time comes to apply, so careful record keeping of any such transactions is required. The maximum period of disqualification is limited to thirty-six months (or sixty months for transfers into a trust), from the date the money is transferred. It can be a shorter period of time if less than the maximum is given away. If a period of ineligibility is created, under no circumstances should one make application for Medicaid until expiration of that period or serious consequences may be triggered. As part of the application process, family records will be scrutinized for up to thirty-six months before the date of application. It is important that family members begin to keep detailed records of all expenditures in anticipation of this review. A rough guideline would be documentation for any expenditure over $500, but this is only a rule of thumb. Medicaid reserves the right to scrutinize an expense of any amount.

Some transfers are exempt for Medicaid purposes. If a child has been living at home for two years or more with the principal goal of taking care of the FTD parent so that he or she can remain within the community, that gift would not have any effect on the Medicaid eligibility process. However, one must have a POA that authorizes such transactions when parents cannot take this action themselves.

Excluded Assets

Some assets are exempt and some assets can be declared "unavailable"—which is essentially the same, since those assets are not counted. Rules don't exist for each and every asset that exists. The way something gets counted can be open to interpretation. States may count assets in different ways. There can even be variations within a state depending on how one Medicaid office interprets the rules versus another. In some states, an Individual Retirement Account (or any other type of qualified retirement plan, such as a 401k) owned by the community spouse is exempt. Unless the assets are minimal and simple, an Elder Care lawyer should be retained. Such attorneys can develop a plan for addressing these highly complex issues based on the assets and the requirements of their particular state.

The primary asset that is excluded in all states is the residence in which the community spouse resides. If the family member being institutionalized is single and the family wishes to retain his residence for his possible return, they can. However, because of a change in the Medicaid laws, which now provides for an estate recovery program, the state would place a lien on the property. Therefore, if your family member lives alone and he cannot remain at home, the house should be sold.

If the house is not sold, the Medicaid Estate Recovery lien is calculated based upon the amount of money that Medicaid has paid under the program. However, this amount is only assessed against the probate estate in some states, and against any asset (including nonprobate assets, such as a jointly owned residence) in other states. This lien is then considered along with your family member's other creditors and satisfied from those remaining assets. Again, this applies only if the family member is single. If he is married, the residence of the community spouse is untouched (as long as the title to the house is in the name of the surviving spouse only or, if jointly owned, the title is with right of survivorship or tenants in the entirety).

OTHER OPTIONS

Sometimes families are committed to keeping their loved one at home. This is not always possible for everyone, since the costs can be staggering. There are a couple of options for freeing up assets to help cover the costs. These options deplete the assets of the family and should only be pursued as a last resort. If the homeowner is sixty-five or over, it is possible to get a reverse mortgage. This frees up the equity in the home while allowing the person to continue to live there. Some mortgage holders limit the amount of equity available to be drawn upon. When the person (and her spouse, if married) dies (or, if not married, transfers to a nursing home), ownership of the house goes to the bank holding the reverse mortgage. Any equity that is left goes to the beneficiaries. If the equity gets used up, the person (and spouse) can still remain in the home for as long as they live.

Another option is to draw on any life insurance the person may have. Some policies sold in the last ten years have what is called an "accelerated death benefit." Under this provision, the insurance company will advance a portion of death proceeds (usually around 70 percent) for use by the insured. The remainder is then payable to the beneficiary upon death. Generally this cannot be exercised until the person has only six or twelve months to live. The time allowed varies between insurance companies. If the policy does not have this provision, there are independent companies who will "buy" the policy and name themselves as the beneficiary and advance a portion of the death benefit. The insurance company then assumes responsibility for all future premiums. Generally, they don't have limits on how long the person is expected to live before they will do this. In return for taking the risk that the individual will live a long time, they keep the remainder. Sometimes this can be as much as 50 percent or more of the death benefit. This device is called a "viatical settlement." See your insurance agent as well as an Elder Care lawyer for advice before entering into any such controversial agreement.

CONCLUSION

The legal and financial issues for a family dealing with FTD are formidable. There are no easy answers. What there is, is a complex maze of programs and legalities to be faced. Unfortunately, our healthcare system is based on a medical model, not one suited to dementia, let alone a form of dementia most healthcare providers have not dealt with before. It is like fitting a square peg into a round hole. Family members are strongly encouraged to seek help from legal and financial professionals familiar with the issues described in this chapter.

Many of the issues are filled with technicalities. One misstep can cause delays, angst, and sometimes thousands of dollars. For instance, failure to spend down to below $89,300 by even one dollar can mean a delay of up to a month before qualifying for Medicaid. This can mean a month of several thousands of dollars of additional nursing home costs that must be paid by the family.

Many of these issues are governed at the state level (and sometimes can even vary within a state from county to county, district to district). This presents a compelling reason to engage a knowledge-able professional familiar with your area. Finally, some things like a living will and record keeping in anticipation of filing for Medicaid need to be undertaken as soon as possible.

Hopefully this chapter has provided the necessary signposts for caregivers to make their way through the maze.

RESOURCES

To locate an Elder Care lawyer near you, contact:

- *Local Bar Association.* Check your local telephone directory or conduct an Internet search for this information.
- *National Academy of Elder Care Lawyers.* 520-881-4005, www.naela.com.
- *National Association of State Medicaid Directors.* http://medicaid.aphsa. org/default.htm, click on "links" to get state Medicaid Web sites.

Part IV
Caring for Yourself

CHAPTER 22

A Daily Break:

Respite and Personal Care for the Caregiver

VIVIAN E. GREENBERG

UNDERSTANDING CAREGIVING

"**C**aregiving" and "caregiver" are just about household terms today. There are books and conferences for caregivers. There are support groups for caregivers. And there are organizations like the National Family Caregiver's Association that advocate and lobby for them. In 1998, New Jersey Governor Christine Whitman established an Eldercare Committee to study the needs and status of caregivers. Because people are living longer, with more chronic and disabling illness, all this public awareness is a good thing. Unless caregivers take care of themselves, paying attention to their own needs for emotional and physical well-being, they will, to quote Boen Hallum of the Central Ohio Parkinson Society, "become an extinct species." And then, who will be left to take care of the increasing numbers of elderly and disabled?

While the words "caregiver" and "caregiving" basically describe what the job is all about, they do not do justice to the range of emotions that flood the caregiver. Almost academic in tone, these words seems to convey the message that giving care is some kind of cerebral exercise. Just *know* what to do, and the caregiver will be okay. Not so!

Caregiving is a complex process. It is a mixture of dark and light emotions that are normal. The guilt, the shame, the anger, the sadness, the confusion, and powerlessness that surface at one time or another come with the territory. Caregivers need to know this crucial fact. They need to know, as well, that in no way does harboring these feelings indicate that they are bad people or poor caregivers.

What these darker emotions accomplish, however, is to create stress and to obscure the lighter emotions that caregiving does hold. The *joy* of making a difference in someone's life, the *competence* of being able to do things you thought you could never do, and the *empowerment* of learning the healthcare system lose their value in the wake of darker emotions.

Caregivers, eager to provide the best care possible to the person they love, all too frequently forget that they too have a life that must be lived and interests and dreams that should be pursued. It is not unusual that in their zeal to be the best and do it all, they lose their own personal identity, not only becoming an extension of the person they care for, but becoming ill themselves. The line they tread between self and other is a fine and slippery one.

What caregivers—and all of us—should be taught in our moral and religious lessons is that self-love is considerably different from selfishness or self-centeredness. Or as Shakespeare so eloquently put it in his drama *Henry V,* "Self love is not so vile a sin as self neglect."

All caregiving is hard and stressful. In caring for someone with FTD, the challenges are different and perhaps even more exasperating. The three crucial elements that make caregiving the trial it is are: (1) The unpredictability of the patient's behavior, in that the caregiver has no idea what will trigger it; (2) The bizarre nature of the behavior itself—lack of inhibition, compulsivity, aggression, or impulsiveness; (3) The lack of empathy and emotion in the patient, which on a daily basis can leave the caregiver feeling demoralized, unappreciated, and irrelevant.

Given the presence of these factors, caregivers of FTD patients are at high risk for depression, moodiness, sleeplessness, and chronic anxiety plus physical ailments like high blood pressure, gastrointestinal problems, back ache, and chronic pain. The energy involved both in being on constant alert for the triggers of inappropriate behaviors and in managing them once they happen is enough to wipe out ten caregivers, let alone one. How, for example, does one deal with someone who is compelled to wash his hands or brush his teeth every hour? Or someone who is compelled to walk around in circles? What must it be like for the caregiver that must constantly walk on eggshells because she is never quite sure when she will be embarrassed by some inappropriate action or word?

And, as if all of the above were not enough to burn out the most capable caregiver, consider how painful it is to care for someone whose emotional range is a flat line. How does one relate to a person on a daily basis who cannot register a smile, a laugh, or a tad of excitement? How does one relate to someone whose mood cannot be figured out because his facial expression is always the same?

Add to this cauldron of stress the fact that the person who is being cared for is not the person he once was. Behaviors, attitudes, affect, and values are opposite of what they were. It is as if the person you once lived with and had a relationship with is now a stranger. It is as if that earlier person is dead. You may find yourself crying a lot, either in anger or grief.

The fact is that you are mourning, grieving for the loss of the person you once knew. The anger and grief are normal. They must have an outlet for expression, else they will weigh you down in bitterness and remorse. Friends help, but grief counseling is better. The point is, you must get support! Remember too that it is okay to punch pillows, cry, and talk to others, as much as you need to. To deny the grief or to push away the feelings by being perpetually busy will not take you through the process to the other side, where you can feel release and acceptance.

WHAT IS RESPITE?

All caregivers must get respite. Defined literally, "respite" means a short interval of rest or relief. Since each of us is different in habits, tastes, and interests, what is respite for one may not be respite for the other. Consequently, sources of respite are varied. Some of the more common are:

- taking a walk
- visiting friends
- sitting at a café with a newspaper and coffee
- working out at a gym
- playing cards or games like bridge or checkers

- sports, like tennis, bowling, shooting baskets, and golfing
- meditation
- dancing
- lunching with friends
- movies with friends

Other caregivers report that respite for them is watching the sunset or the leaves fall, being with grandchildren, going to the library, or shopping. Whatever relaxes or brings peace of mind or physical or mental enjoyment to the caregiver is respite.

Of note, as well, is that your area office on aging has funds for caregiver respite. Each county has different eligibility requirements, so call to find out what they are. In addition, the National Family Caregivers Association (800-896-3650) in Kensington, Maryland, offers information and referral services for respite services nation-wide. While the costs of home care are frequently high, you must remember that those who come to help out serve *two* people—not just the patient but the caregiver, too.

Caregivers must escape from the confinement and isolation of providing care. For caregivers of FTD patients, however, being with others is a number-one imperative. A chat room on the computer may be helpful, but it is not enough. Caregivers must get out and be with people they can see, touch, talk to, and hear. Human connection is what will make them feel they have a life and identity outside of the world of caregiving. Human connection will give their lives meaning and purpose.

It is not surprising that results of studies on caregivers of FTD patients suggest that when caregivers early on pay attention to their needs for social support and respite, not only is their quality of life enhanced but also that of the patient. Indeed, institutionalization may even be delayed.

What it all comes down to, again to quote Boen Hallum, is that "what is good for the caregiver will be ultimately good for the patient."[1] If the caregiver is replenished, she will have more within her to give. She will return to her caregiving duties a more patient and more empathic caregiver.

Edward M. Hallowell, M.D., author of *Connection* and professor of psychiatry at Harvard Medical School, tells us that connection is the single most important factor in having a satisfying life. The

unique and healing comforts of connection cannot be found any-
where else. He goes on to state that social isolation is a higher predictor of death than the commonly accepted dangers of cigarettes,
obesity, and high cholesterol. That frequency of visits with friends
and number of meetings attended (social, religious, political) are
what create contentment and meaning in life. That human connection, being with others, has the magical property to make us feel
better.

KNOWING WHEN YOU NEED RESPITE

The big question remaining is: How do you know when you need
respite? Ideally, of course, respite should be thought about and put
into place before a crisis happens. Home health aides, neighbors,
friends, and daycare programs should all be known about and put
into use. A network of support services should be at your fingertips:
names and numbers all posted on the refrigerator. This, however, is
rarely the case.

The signs of stress are not bashful about making themselves
known, but caregivers often deny or ignore their persistent messages. One caregiver said that she thought she was managing just
fine, until her dentist told her she was grinding down her teeth in
her sleep. Another thought she needed no help whatsoever until she
started falling asleep in her car on the way home from work. Yet
another, who was referred for counseling by her dermatologist, suffered from a stress-related eczema characterized by itching redness
and inflammation.

Other stress-related disorders are: headaches, back aches,
stomach problems, and high blood pressure. Depression and anxiety
run rampant among those giving care to loved ones. Inability to
sleep, poor appetite, and loss of energy are symtoms of depression.
Inability to concentrate and panic attacks, characterized by rapid
heart beat and fast breathing, are some of the signs of anxiety.

Although caregivers may not know when they are edging into
the terrain of burn-out, the persons they are caring for will. Irritability, impatience, resentment, shortness of temper, the feeling that
"I'd rather be anyplace but here," all will effect the caregiving relationship. When care is not being given with a full heart, the patient

knows that something is not right. The patient knows the caregiver isn't emotionally there. And it is that "quality," in contrast to "quantity," of care that matters most.

Remember, the effectiveness of your caregiving is in direct proportion to its quality. The underpinning of quality care cannot be anger, guilt, or resentment.

Caregivers, you must take care of yourselves! Eat well, get enough sleep, and push yourself to exercise. A fifteen-minute walk every day can make an enormous difference in your mood and attitude. Rent a movie that will make you laugh and laugh and laugh some more. Norman Cousins, in his uplifting book, *Anatomy of an Illness*, has proven to us that laughter is the magic potion to heal ailing minds and bodies.

So, FTD caregivers, get out there! You are valuable people, first to yourselves, then to your patient. Don't forget who you are. You will lose control over your lives, and become resentful caregivers. So visit friends, play cards, go to meetings and luncheons. Gather "warm fuzzies" wherever you can. You, more than anyone, know about the cruel tricks life can play. There's not a minute to lose!

NOTE

1. Boen Hallum, *Parkinson's Disease: A Caregiver's Observation* (Columbus: Central Ohio Parkinson Society, 1998).

CHAPTER 23

From Loss to Life:

Managing Emotions and Grief

REV. DAVID COTTON

"I just can't stand to see him suffer like that!" How many times have we heard someone utter those words about a loved one? They seem so common that we don't really even stop to consider what is really being said. "*I* can't stand to see her suffer like that." The pain of illness is *plural pain*. The ripple effect of illness reaches out from patient to spouse to children to family to friends to colleagues, and on and on in ever widening circles. Family and friends experience pain just like the patient, sometimes even more. As chaplain in an acute-care hospital, I often hear family members exclaim that they can't bear to see their loved one suffer. When the patient is either sedated or comatose, the only real suffering is on the part of those who are caregivers.

When the illness is FTD, the stakes are even higher than with other physical ailments, because the situation is more complicated. The pain experienced by family and friends of the patient is the pain of grief. We must be willing to let go of the notion that grieving means that a person has died. Grieving results from loss, and yes, from the *little deaths* that loss introduces into our lives.

LOSS ALONG THE WAY

Caregivers of those with FTD are faced with a devastating array of losses with which they must learn to cope if they are to survive the onslaught of this progressive, incurable disease. Their loved one is still there, still a part of life in the relationship and the family, but he is not the same. The dramatic changes in personality have the effect of making the patient a different person, sometimes gradually, sometimes rapidly, before the very eyes of those closest. The first significant loss which must be grieved, then, is the loss of self—the loss of the person who used to be there before the condition took that self away and created a new personality and a new person inside the same body.

From witty and communicative to nonverbal, from socially adept to totally uninhibited, from intelligent and productive to irrational and disinterested, from caring and compassionate to angry and self-centered, frontotemporal dementia is the insidious destruction of a person and the unwelcome appearance of a new one. Having a different person in the same body, in the same relationship, can be very confusing and disorienting to the caregiver. This is especially true when the disease comes on so slowly and subtly that it is difficult to tell whether the change is due to emotional and psychological changes instead of physical deterioration of the brain. Often, irritation and resentment can build in response to personality changes. These feelings can sometimes germinate long before the caregiver's awareness and understanding that their loved ones changes are due to FTD. These changes are not the product of negative attitudes or emotions and not the fault of the FTD sufferer. The result may be a sense of guilt over the expression of anger or frustration when it is realized that the cause was physical and not emotional. This guilt often mixes with the inevitable sadness at losing someone while she is still physically present.

The caregiver, having lost the person who used to be there, in turn grieves the second loss—the loss of the relationship that used to exist. The conversation that used to be so meaningful is no longer possible. The emotional support of a trusted spouse is gone. Physical intimacy, once so important, is no longer present. The social life as a couple is over for good. The spouse as caregiver has lost not only a person, but also a partner.

This loss, though, is not limited to the marriage relationship. Parents see the order of the world turned upside down when they must bid good-bye to the child they know and love while that child is still alive! Siblings lose a part of their lives, someone who "was always supposed to be there," and siblings are forced to face their own mortality and vulnerability as they wonder, "Am I next?" Friends and coworkers, too, face the reality of loss as they see the familiar and the comfortable slip away, only to be replaced by confusion and awkwardness. All relationships are impacted by the losses caused by frontotemporal dementia.

Grieving the loss of the relationship carries with it strong feelings of loneliness and isolation. The first person you greet in the morning, the one you seek out for advice and approval, the one with whom you share everything, the person with whom you fell in love is gone, and no one else feels it like you do. The sense of isolation becomes even deeper when the caregiver realizes that so few people understand even the basics of FTD. This lack of understanding often results in faulty comparisons with and improper identification of frontotemporal dementia as Alzheimer's disease, leading to further frustration and isolation.

Perhaps an equally difficult third loss is the loss of personal freedom for caregivers. They may need to quit their jobs in order to adequately care for their loved one. Time away from home is limited by the constant demands of caregiving. Networks of friends and acquaintances break down as the caregiver is swallowed up more and more by increasing responsibilities. This loss of personal freedom can lead to feelings of anger as the question, "Why me?" inevitably arises. And then the guilt usually is not far behind as images of selfishness descend upon the psyche of the caregiver.

Economic considerations engender a fourth experience of loss as well. The earning power of the person with FTD is lost; at the same time, the financial demands for professional assistance are on the rise. The loss of the status quo is a present reality, and the loss of the future that had been planned and dreamed of sends the ripples of loss far into the course of time.

OWNING YOUR GRIEF

So how do caregivers cope with this nightmarish collection of losses? How can they deal with the grief that washes over them and threatens to sweep them away? First, caregivers must "own their grief" and accept it as an integral part of the experience they are facing. Owning our grief means allowing ourselves to feel sad, to feel discouraged, and yes, even to feel sorry for ourselves. Owning our grief means that we are willing to accept that each person's grieving has elements of similarity, but that each person's grief is unique, to time, personality, circumstances, and so many other factors which make feelings so difficult to quantify and put into a formula.

Owning our grief means that we learn not to feel guilty about grieving and that we understand grieving not as right or wrong, proper or improper. Grief is just an uninvited yet omnipresent companion with caregivers on the journey of caring for one who suffers from FTD. And owning our grief means that we do not allow anyone else to *make* us feel guilty, intentionally or unintentionally. No one understands, no one *can* understand the pain of dealing with this disease. You can describe your nightmare to someone else, but no one is capable of experiencing the emotions that are yours and yours alone. This is especially true for a nightmare from which you never wake up.

This journey of care and grief does not flow on a steady or predictable curve. There are no reliable stages through which we must move. As caregivers, it is crucial that we not place arbitrary timetables and limits on our feelings of grief over the losses we have sustained. "It's been three months, six months, or six years; the number doesn't matter! I or you should be done with the crying and grieving by now and moving on with life." We all hear messages like this, both from ourselves and from those around us.

Owning our grief means affirming our own individual timetable, which, as mentioned above, is not a steady curve. Grief is much more like a roller coaster ride than a climb up an inclined plane. FTD caregivers are especially aware of this. They are facing the reality of adjusting to the their loved one's changed behaviors and lost abilities, only to wake up and find that those behaviors and abilities have changed again, necessitating a new set of coping strategies and skills. Each loss brings with it the companion of grief. The only way to survive that grief is to own it and face it and hold on for whatever lies around the next curve.

Owning our grief reaches past ourselves and enters the lives of those around us, recognizing that they too are grieving. Children, brothers and sisters, parents, friends and colleagues; all feel the loss of the person they knew. As a practitioner, experience has confirmed that often the most difficult aspect for grieving families is the capacity to allow others to grieve in their own distinct way. Unfortunately, the first impulse is to judge that others are not grieving appropriately if their expression and experience do not match our own. As we learned that grief is unique to us, so we must allow each person affected by the loss to grieve in his individual way. We can own *our* grief by allowing others the right to own *theirs*.

A Child's Grief

Children certainly face some aspects of grieving that are particular to their situation. One important issue is the role reversal between parent and child. As the patient's abilities for self-care decline, the children find themselves more and more in the role of parent for one who should be caring for them. The resulting confusion and perhaps anger may produce feelings of guilt and resentment. It is important to be sensitive to their needs during this time and to give them permission to own their feelings.

As the disease progresses and inhibitions fall away, bizarre behavior may result in embarrassment for younger children of an FTD sufferer. Children may withdraw or vent their anger and frustration at the primary caregiver. This is a time to call in outside resources to assist in dealing with the panoply of emotions that accompany having a parent with FTD. If children are in school, be sure to notify administration, teachers, and counselors so they are aware of the situation at home and can be sensitive to changes in affect or behavior. In addition, a counselor from outside the family can be extremely helpful because the children will have the freedom to express frustrations that they may not share with a close family member who is also grieving.

There may be problems at school due to a number of reasons. Children experiencing such basic, life-changing upheavals at home may question the priority and importance adults put on grades, homework, and school attendance, no matter whether they are in elementary school or graduate school. Children's sense of priorities may be drastically affected by the loss of the parent they once knew and depended upon. Readjustment will require patient listening and measured reactions that stress the importance of maintaining a life separate from the reality of the disease.

One source of difficulty with children is the question of how much information to share. Do they need to know everything? Will they just be weighed down even more by the burden of dealing with the details? Each situation is different and varies with family dynamics, ages of the children, personalities, etc., but in general it is best to share the truth as much as possible.

Often, when the truth is shared, the response from the children is either silence or far less than had been anticipated. What's the answer? Listen, listen, and listen some more. Give them time to collect their thoughts. Give them permission to be mixed up and reaffirm that you want to hear what they are thinking and feeling even if they don't understand it themselves. Don't assume you know what they are thinking and feeling. Open yourself up and share your feelings with them. It's the best way to make them feel comfortable that they can trust you with their feelings.

The loss and reaction to it are different but just as devastating for older children. In their late teens and twenties, the establishment of an adult relationship with their parents is a major accomplishment. Yet for those who have a parent suffering from FTD, the entire process is short-circuited. Older children may have a distorted impression of their responsibilities in the face of serious illness and may feel the need to "fix" the situation.

At this age level, plans are put on hold and lives are interrupted at just the time when they were supposed to blossom in independence and self-sufficiency. Their wings are put away for later, their role becomes caregiver (for both parents), the resentment inevitably surfaces, and the resulting guilt can be devastating and debilitating. Older children still need their parents, and their reaction to loss must not be underestimated.

A Parent's Grief

For the parents of an FTD sufferer, the world has been turned upside down. A child with neurodegenerative illness—this is not the way things are supposed to work! Anger and fear collide as thoughts and feelings tumble around inside. Parents and other family members may stay away in order to hide feelings they are ashamed to admit are present. Visits may be short, and conversation may revolve around meaningless topics unrelated to the situation. However frustrating this behavior may be, patience and tolerance are the order of the day. Confrontations will only result in driving family members farther away. Honest sharing of one's own struggles and conflicting emotions may be the best prescription for opening up parents and other family members to face their feelings and own their grief.

Declaring War and Calling in the Reserves

Finally, owning our grief means admitting that we need help and seeking that help wherever it can be found. Recently in the intensive care unit here at the hospital, I was with a family when the doctor came to talk with them about the sudden onset of a life-threatening condition. "We are now at war!" the physician exclaimed to the family, assuring them that all resources at our disposal would be thrown into the battle when and if needed.

As a primary caregiver for someone with FTD, it's time to declare war and call out the reserves. *When people offer to assist in a particular way*, let them! Have a list of helpful jobs from which they can choose when people say, "If there's something I can do. . . ." It's normal to want to do everything yourself, but why should you? Your family and friends love you and care about you, and they want to be a part of this area of your life. They want to reach out to help the patient and help you. The battle is huge and the stakes are high. *This is the time to muster all the forces you can to give you some time to sleep, some time to get out of the house, some time to care for yourself.* (For more information see chapter 20.)

FOUR STEPS TO EMOTIONAL HEALTH

How does one move through the rough, rocky, uneven terrain of grief and along toward emotional health? Consider this four-step model, a process that will not only enable caregivers to survive the experience of facing FTD, but will also empower them to grow stronger and more confident. The four steps to emotional health are *reimage, refocus, remember,* and *refresh.*

I. Reimage

This requires the caregiver to move from what used to be to what is, from what should be to what *can be*. There is a powerful urge to avoid the reality of the new situation and to expend a great deal of time and energy trying to maintain the illusion that things can still be the way they used to be. *To reimage is to let go of the desire to live in the past and to face the present with open eyes and an open mind, accepting the truth.* You are loving someone, living with someone, looking at someone who has become somebody else. This requires a tremendous supply of courage to keep going forward.

No, it's not fair that FTD has invaded your loved one, your family, your life. Life should be different, but life is not about "should." Life just is. Reimaging calls us to live in the now. It is difficult to put away the dreams of what should be, but living in the present is liberating and freeing. Reimaging allows us to appreciate the beauty of today. It calls us to see the good, to find the humor, to appreciate the blessing of a phone call from a friend, the gift of a radiant sunset, the delicacy of a rose, the brightness of a smile. Reimaging is the foundation for future growth that each of the next three steps can build upon.

2. Refocus

Caring for a loved one with FTD can become such an overwhelming job that one's entire life is swallowed up, and the disease becomes the only thing in sight. Refocusing calls upon the caregiver to see past the disease. First, it is important to remember that the disease and the person are different and distinct. We must learn to focus on the person, seeing so much more than the disease.

In the same way, caregivers are called to look past the disease and see themselves apart from its ravages. Caregivers, too, run the risk of defining their own lives by the disease, allowing it to shape and fashion them as it has the victim. The caregiver, then, becomes a secondary victim. Refocusing beckons us to see our lives and to see ourselves as so much bigger than any disease. Of course, FTD is a segment of our life, and its impact is profound. But emotional health comes when we refocus and see the big picture of life where there is health as well as disease, courage as well as fear, stability as well as unpredictability, laughter as well as tears, faith as well as doubt. It's what we choose to focus on that creates the picture of our life. Refocusing means realizing that there is a choice and that only we can make it. *To refocus is to choose the positive, the good, and the healthy as our focal points and to train our eyes and our hearts to see the good amid the bad.*

3. Remember

Even though it may seem that FTD has stolen a person away from you, there is so much that the disease cannot touch, so much it cannot take from you, unless you let it! FTD cannot take away the past, the precious memories of time you once shared. It cannot take away the love you experience, the love that will last a lifetime. This ugly disease cannot take away your faith, in God and in yourself, faith that there is a power so much greater than this or any disease, faith that you can not only survive, but overcome. Give yourself permission to remember the good times you shared: how you met, important life transitions, times of laughter and lightness. *Remember what brought you to where you are now, and savor the precious memories.*

4. Refresh

The essence of refreshing is taking care of yourself. It's so easy to become consumed with caregiving for another, that caregiving for yourself gets neglected or left behind altogether. *Refresh calls us to create an oasis of health in the midst of the desert of disease.*

How do we create an oasis? First, we need to get help. The FTD caregiver needs professional, physical, emotional, and spiritual assistance to make the soul a place that blossoms and grows. Sometimes the obstacles to obtaining professional help may seem overwhelming. Insurance is reluctant to pay for help in the home and notoriously unwilling to pay for professional counseling for the caregiver. But don't be discouraged! Home nursing, home health aides to assist with personal care, social workers, etc. may not be offered, but they often are available to those willing to negotiate the tortuous route of paperwork and red tape. Therapy for the caregiver is not at the top of most insurance companies' list of necessary provisions, but for the determined, persistence often can bring the payoff of a specific number of paid sessions with a professional counselor or therapist. Ask a friend to help with the insurance forms and phone calls instead of feeling you have to do it all yourself.

If at the end of the process you find you cannot procure the services of professionals, don't give up. Refreshment can be found in other places as well. Be creative. Check with your local congregation to see if it sponsors volunteers who might come to your home to help with care or to give you some time away from the demands of caregiving. Consult with a local dementia organization or support group chapter to obtain information on assistance available in your area. If you can't afford professional therapy, check to see if there is a group of other caregivers with whom you can meet and share your experiences while learning from the journeys of others. Sometimes it's comforting to know that others are facing the same trials and troubles that you are, even if they don't have all the answers. (For more information on support networks, see chapter 20.)

In addition, refresh means that you are willing to acknowledge that you need practical, physical help. This is the time to call on extended family, friends, neighbors, congregants—whoever can give you a helping hand. Raking the leaves, cleaning the gutters, mowing the lawn, shoveling the walk, fixing a lamp, etc., these are the chores which detract from your quality of life when caregiving prevents you from getting around to them. Others may not be comfortable with providing direct patient care, and you may not be comfortable with that either. But there are many people in your circle of family and friends who would be willing to assist you with a specific job, either as a one-time help or on a regular basis. They win, you win, and your loved one wins. Others ease their frustration and feelings of helplessness by pitching in. You are able to find time for yourself to relax and to refresh your body, mind, and soul. Your loved one has the benefit of your being able to spend more concentrated "together time" instead of being pulled away by so many distractions. Let go, and let others help!

A seminary professor of mine once said, "Life is what you do with fifteen minutes." This statement has had a profound effect on my life, as I have realized and have helped others to realize that refresh doesn't have to mean a vacation to the tropics or even a day at the spa. *Refresh can and does mean grabbing a few moments of peace and tranquillity when you can.* It means intentionally making time for emotional rest and relaxation, building these times into the day where and when you can.

As a caregiver for someone with FTD, of course the opportunities for a vacation in the traditional sense of the word are few and far between, if not impossible. To refresh, however, is to believe in and to practice the art of the possible. A cup of tea in the sunshine, a daily devotional reading, writing a journal entry, praying or meditating in a designated spot, walking in the yard or the garden, calling a friend for support. These are opportunities to refresh yourself. *Taking time for yourself is not selfish.* On the contrary, times of refreshment will make you a better caregiver because you will be more patient and more able to handle the next crisis, which will inevitably arise. Take fifteen minutes for yourself . . . and refresh!

In addition to body and mind, refresh applies to the spirit, to the soul. It's so tempting to look at this time of caregiving as merely a time of destruction: of a person, of a relationship, of a dream. But this time can also be a period of creation, a time of development for your soul and your relationship to God. The Judeo-Christian tradition recognizes the concept of *shalom*, a word that is normally translated as "peace," but which signifies so much more. The truer, deeper meaning involves health and, perhaps even more fully, may be described as wholeness.

Wholeness, completeness, how can this be possible when you are losing someone? To answer this question, we must step outside ourselves and turn for answers to something greater than ourselves, something greater than the problem, greater than the disease. If you are religious, the structures are already in place. Consult your clergy and make him/her a part of the solution. Seek out spiritual resources in books, tapes, even on television. Find out if your local congregation sponsors prayer groups, support groups, study groups, etc. that will get you in touch with others who share your faith and who can share your journey with you and pray for you.

Feelings of anger or disappointment with God are natural at a time such as this. I tell people with whom I work that it's okay to have those feelings, for a time. "It's an okay place to visit, but you don't want to live there," is my phrase. If you are religious, if you have been religious, don't try to fight this battle without the strength and courage and power and peace that only your faith and your God can provide. The prophet Isaiah talks of God's redeeming acts as bringing "times of refreshing," and these times can be yours, too. Just reach out.

All persons are not religious, but all are spiritual. If you fall into this category, don't neglect the spirituality that can bring wholeness and health. Don't be afraid to take time to look inside, to go deep into your secret, spiritual places to find the meaning that this life event holds for you. Merely operating on a surface level will never get you to the places where your spirit can bring you peace and tranquillity. Just as it is important to go inside, it is equally critical to go outside yourself. Look beyond yourself to a higher power in order to gain perspective, which we cannot have from our point of view in the midst of the problem. Allow your spirit to probe deeply inside and to soar unfettered outside, and you will find where you need to go the next time you need to refresh.

SEEING THE WHOLE

Perhaps you may be wondering whether you will ever get over the trauma of caring for and ultimately losing someone who is a victim of FTD. In many years of counseling with hundreds of families facing grief and loss, I can assure you that you need not worry about "getting over it." That isn't the task you must complete. Instead of getting over it, which seems impossible because it is, those who are experiencing a great loss need to "get on with it."

"Getting on with it" simply means getting on with life: as it is, each minute, each hour, each day. Getting on with life involves "owning your grief" as you learn that loss is a component of your life and the lives of those close to you and to your loved one.

A friend completing her master's degree in art from New York University used a unique perspective for her final show. Every work of art she produced, from canvases to plaster figures to metal sculptures, had a hole in it. But instead of being just an empty space, the hole was incorporated into each work of art so that the hole was part of the whole. And the whole was still beautiful!

Living with grief and loss is a daily exercise in living life with a hole in it. Through "owning our grief" and through seeking emotional, physical, and spiritual health in the fourfold plan of reimage, refocus, remember, and refresh, we can see life as bigger than the hole left by frontotemporal dementia. We can learn to see the beauty of life again, the beauty of the whole.

Contributing
Authors

Chapter 1

Martin Rosser, M.A., M.D., F.R.C.P.
Head of Dementia Research Group
Institute of Neurology
Queen Square, London, United Kingdom

Chapter 2

Murray Grossman, M.D., Ed.D.
Associate Professor of Neurology and Psychiatry
Department of Neurology
University of Pennsylvania Medical Center
Philadelphia, Pennsylvania

Chapter 3

Jennifer Farmer, M.S., C.G.C.
Genetic Counselor/Research Coordinator
Center for Neurodegenerative Disease Research
University of Pennsylvania
Philadelphia, Pennsylvania

Chapter 4

Carol F. Lippa, M.D.
Professor and Chief, MCP Neurology

Director, Memory Disorders Center
Drexel University College of Medicine
Philadelphia, Pennsylvania

Chapter 5
Tiffany W. Chow, M.D.
Clinician Scientist
Rotman Research Institute
Toronto, Ontario, Canada

Chapter 6
Keith M. Robinson, M.D.
Chief, Division of Rehabilitation Medicine
Department of Rehabilitation Medicine
Pennsylvania Hospital
Associate Professor of Rehabilitation Medicine
University of Pennsylvania
Philadelphia, Pennsylvania

Chapter 7
Carol F. Lippa, M.D.
Professor and Chief, MCP Neurology
Director, Memory Disorders Center
Drexel University College of Medicine
Philadelphia, Pennsylvania

Chapter 8
Jennifer Farmer, M.S., C.G.C.
Genetic Counselor/Research Coordinator
Center for Neurodegenerative Disease Research
University of Pennsylvania
Philadelphia, Pennsylvania

Virginia M.-Y. Lee, Ph.D.
Professor of Pathology and Laboratory Medicine
Director, Center for Neurodegenerative Disease Research
University of Pennsylvania Medical Center
Philadelphia, Pennsylvania

John Q. Trojanowski, M.D., Ph.D.
Professor of Pathology and Laboratory Medicine
Director, Institute on Aging at Penn
Codirector, Center for Neurodegenerative Disease Research
University of Pennsylvania School of Medicine
Philadelphia, Pennsylvania

Chapter 9

Jordan Grafman, Ph.D.
Chief, Cognitive Neuroscience Section
National Institute of Neurological Disorders and Stroke
National Institute of Health
Bethesda, Maryland

Chapter 10

Erica Wollman, M.Ed., C.C.C.-S.L.P.
Clinical specialist in speech language pathology
Department of Otorhinolaryngology
University of Pennsylvania Medical Center
Philadelphia, Pennsylvania

Chapter 11

Heather J. Cianci, P.T., G.C.S.
The Dan Aaron Parkinson's Rehabilitation Center
The Penn Neurological Institute
Philadelphia, Pennsylvania

Chapter 12

Lisa Ann Fagan, O.T.R./L., C.A.L.A.
Rehabilitation and assisted-living management consultant
Adjunct Instructor, Department of Occupational Therapy
Philadelphia University
Hatboro, Pennsylvania

Chapter 13

Lisa Ann Fagan, O.T.R./L., C.A.L.A.
Rehabilitation and assisted-living management consultant
Adjunct instructor, Department of Occupational Therapy

Philadelphia University
Hatboro, Pennsylvania

Chapter 14
Lisa Ann Fagan, O.T.R./L., C.A.L.A.
Rehabilitation and assisted-living management consultant
Adjunct instructor, Department of Occupational Therapy
Philadelphia University
Hatboro, Pennsylvania

Chapter 15
Katherine P. Rankin, Ph.D.
Assistant Professor of Neuropsychology
Memory and Aging Center
Department of Neurology
University of California San Francisco
San Francisco, California

Chapter 16
Bruce L. Miller, M.D.
Clausen Distinguished Professor of Neurology
Director, Memory and Aging Center
Department of Neurology
University of California San Francisco
San Francisco, California
Medical Director, John Douglas French Foundation for
    Alzheimer's Disease

Rosalie Gearhart, R.N., M.S., C.S.
Clinical nurse specialist
Memory and Aging Center
Department of Neurology
University of California San Francisco School of Medicine
Assistant Clinical Professor
University of California San Francisco School of Nursing
San Francisco, California

Chapter 17

Jeannette Castellane, L.S.W.
Social worker, Certified in Gerontology
Luther Crest Retirement Community
Member, Board of Directors, The Ethics Institute and Nexus for
    Geriatric Planning
Allentown, Pennsylvania

Chapter 18

Judy L. Fisher, R.N., M.S., Ph.D. candidate
Chief Executive Officer
HomeCare & HospiceCare of South Jersey
Salem, New Jersey

Susan Riley, C.S.W.
Social worker/Grant coordinator
HomeCare & HospiceCare of South Jersey
Salem, New Jersey

Chapter 19

Morris J. Kaplan, Esq., N.H.A.
Chief Executive Officer
Gwynedd Square Center for Nursing and Convalescent Care
Lansdale, Pennsylvania

Chapter 20

Helen-Ann Comstock
Chair, The Association for Frontotemporal Dementias
Former Pick's disease caregiver, 1978–1984
Executive Director, Alzheimer's Assn. Southeastern Pennsyl-
    vania Chapter, 1985–2000
Philadelphia, Pennsylvania

Chapter 21

Paul L. Feldman, Esq.
Feldman & Feldman
Attorneys at Law
Philadelphia, Pennsylvania
Specializing in Elder Law

Kent S. Jamison, Ph.D.
Vice Chair, The Association for Frontotemporal Dementias
Former caregiver
Consultant to the financial services industry
Former member, Board of Directors, Alzheimer's Assn.
    Northern Connecticut Chapter
Canton, Connecticut

Chapter 22

Vivian E. Greenberg, A.C.S.W., L.C.S.W.
Author, lecturer, consultant, freelance writer, and columnist
Private Practice
Pennington, New Jersey
Specializing in relationships of older adults and their families,
    and issues pertaining to caregiving

Chapter 23

Rev. David Cotton
Coordinator of Pastoral Care
Jersey Shore Medical Center
Neptune, New Jersey

About the Editors

Lisa Radin and her son Gary Radin provided complete care for their husband and father Neil Radin over a four-year period after he was diagnosed with frontotemporal dementia (FTD). Based on this firsthand experience with a devastating and terminal illness, they compiled this collection of expert articles on FTD and dementia. In 1998, following Neil's death, they founded the Neil L. Radin Caregivers Relief Foundation based in New Jersey, and in 1999 were involved in planning the Multidisciplinary Conference on Pick's Disease and Frontotemporal Dementia in Philadelphia. In 2000, Lisa also helped organize the Frontotemporal Dementia and Pick's Disease Criteria Conference at the National Institutes of Health in Bethesda, Maryland. In 2003, she became a founding member of the Association for Frontotemporal Dementias and is currently a special events consultant for the Alzheimer's Association Delaware Valley chapter.

Resources

ADAPTING THE HOME ENVIRONMENT

Abledata, 8630 Fenton St., Ste. 930, Silver Spring, MD 20910, 800-227-0216 (Voice), 301-608-8912 (TTY). www.abledata.com. Database of assistive devices and manufacture/distributor information.

Adaptive Environments Center, 374 Congress St., Ste. 301, Boston, MA 02210, 617-695-1225 (V/TTY), www.adaptenv.org. Home modification resources.

Ageless Design, 12633 159th Court North, Jupiter, FL 33478, 561-745-0210, www.agelessdesign.com. Information on dementia-specific home modifications.

American Association for Retired Persons (AARP), 601 E St., N.W., Washington, DC 20049, 800-424-3410, www.aarp.org. General information about home modifications.

American Occupational Therapy Association, 4720 Montgomery Ln., P.O. Box 31220, Bethesda, MD 20824-1220, 301-652-2682; 800-377-8555 (TDD). www.aota.org. Information on home modification and how to contact an occupational therapist.

LifeEase, P.O. Box 302, Newbury, NH 03255, 800-966-5119 (within USA), or 603-938-5116 (outside of USA), www.lifease.com. Home evaluation information.

National Resource Center on Supportive Housing and Home Modifications, University of Southern California, Andrus Gerontology, www.home-mods.org. Home modification information.

AREA AGENCIES ON AGING (U.S.)

These agencies provide information on local services and Medicaid, and they also provide many helpful services to patients and families. Listings for Area Agencies on Aging are located under "Guide to Human Services" in the blue pages of the telephone book. You must apply for state and federal financial aid (Medicaid) for home care and nursing home care through your local Area Agency on Aging.

CAREGIVER'S ORGANIZATIONS

Family Caregiver Alliance, 690 Market St., Ste. 600, San Francisco, CA, 94104, 415-434-3388, www.caregiver.org. Has a survey of fifteen states' caregiver programs done in 1999: CA, FL, IL, IA, MI, NJ, NY, ND, OH, OR, PA, TX, VA, WA, WI. Fact sheets on various dementias, as well as caregiver issues, statistics, and demographics.

National Family Caregivers Association, 10400 Connecticut Ave., #500, Kensington, MD, 20895-3944, 800-896-3650, www.nfcacares.org. Has a prescription drug discount program for members. Free to join.

Oregon's Caregiving Resource Center, 866-219-7218, www.oregoncare.org. Useful despite the fact that much information may be specific to Oregon. Has a section on legal and financial issues on Web site.

Well Spouse Foundation, 63 W. Main St., Ste. H, Freehold, NJ 07728, 800-838-0879, www.wellspouse.org. Gives support to wives, husbands, and partners of the chronically ill and/or disabled.

EATING UTENSILS AND THICKENERS

AliMed Inc., 297 High St., Dedham, MA   02026, 800-225-2610, www.alimed.com; www.dysphagiatherapy.com. Makes pureed food and has feeding equipment.

Bruce Medical Supplies, 411 Waverly Oaks Rd., Ste. 154, Waltham, MA 02452, 800-225-8446, www.brucemedical.com. Has eating and drinking utensils.

Simply Thick: Phagia-Gel Technologies, LLC., 1374 Clarkson Rd., St. Louis, MO 63011, 800-205-7115, www.simplythick.com. Gel used for thickening foods and drinks.

Thick It: Precision Foods, Inc., 800-333-0003, www.precisionfoods.com. Dry powder used for thickening foods and drinks. Gives link to regional sales representatives. Available at local pharmacies.

ELDER CARE LAWYERS

Elder Care Locator (government web site), 800-677-1116, www.eldercare.gov.
Local Bar Association. Check your local telephone directory or conduct an
Internet search for this information.
National Academy of Elder Care Lawyers, 1604 North Country Club Rd.,
Tucson, AZ 85716, 520-881-4005, www.naela.com.

EXERCISE EQUIPMENT

Over the Door Pulleys: PrePak Products, 4055 Oceanside Blvd., Ste. L,
Oceanside, CA 92056-5821, 800-544-7527, www.prepakproducts.com.
Theraband: KAS Enterprises, 1317 W. 23rd Ave., Covington, LA 70433,
877-860-9534 (toll-free), www.kasenterprises.com/theraband.

GENETICS

Genetic Alliance, Inc., 4301 Connecticut Ave., N.W., Ste. 404, Washington, DC
20008-2304, 202-966-5557, www.geneticalliance.org. Supports individuals with genetic conditions and their families, educates the public, and
advocates for consumer-informed public policies.
National Human Genome Research Institute, National Institutes of Health,
Building 31, Room 4B09, 31 Center Dr., MSC 2152, 9000 Rockville Pike,
Bethesda, MD 20892-2152, 301-402-0911, www.genome.gov. Leads the
Human Genome Project for the National Institutes of Health, conducts
cutting-edge research in its laboratories, and supports genomic science
worldwide. This Web site contains a lot of useful information for the
layperson about the human genome project, genetic research, and genetic
conditions and testing.
National Society of Genetic Counselors, Inc., 233 Canterbury Dr., Wallingford,
PA 19086-6617, 610-872-7608 (voice), www.nsgc.org. Go to Resource Link
to find a genetic counselor.

MEDICAID

National Association of State Medicaid Directors, 810 First St. N.E., Ste. 500,
Washington, DC 20002, 202-682-0100, http://medicaid. aphsa.org/default.
Click on "Links" to get state Medicaid Web site.

MEDICAL CENTERS AND ORGANIZATIONS

If you obtained the diagnosis at a university medical center, you should be able to obtain information from the center. Some centers also offer family consultations and maintain support groups.

Alzheimer's Association (USA), 919 North Michigan Ave., Ste. 1100, Chicago, IL 60611-1676. 800-272-3900 (national helpline), www.alz.org. Maintains local support groups. Publishes a variety of useful brochures (ask for "Related Disorders," among others). The Summer 2001 issue of the Association's *Advances* has an article on frontotemporal dementia, www.alz.org/caregiver/programs/advances.

Alzheimer's Society, United Kingdom, Gordon House, 10 Greencoat Place, London SW1P 1PH, www.alzheimers.org.uk. Ask for the information sheet, "What is fronto-temporal dementia (including Pick's disease)?"

Alzheimer's Australia, P.O. Box 108, Higgins, ACT 2615, Australia, www.alzheimers-org.au. Publishes Help Notes specific to Pick's and a frontal lobe dementia, reading list.

The American Parkinson Disease Association, 1250 Hylan Blvd., Suite 4B, Staten Island, NY 10305-1946, 800-223-2732, www. apdaparkinson.org.

The Association for Frontotemporal Dementias (AFTD), P.O. Box 7191, St. David's, PA 19087-7191. A new nationwide nonprofit organization whose mission is to promote and fund research into finding the cause and cure for frontotemporal dementias; to provide information, education, and support to persons diagnosed with FTD and their families and caregivers; and to educate physicians and allied health professionals about FTD. www.FTD-Picks.org.

Dementia Research Group, United Kingdom, The National Hospital for Neurology and Neurosurgery, Queen Square, London WC1N 3BG, U.K., www.dementia.ion.ucl.ac.uk. Click on CANDID (Counseling ANd Diagnosis In Dementia) for a wealth of information specific to FTD: Pick's disease support group, fact sheets, articles, books, newsletter. Or go directly to CANDID, www.pdsg.uk.

National Hospice Organization, 1901 N. Moore St., Ste. 901, Arlington, VA, 22209, 800-658-8898, www.nho.org.

The National Multiple Sclerosis Society, 733 Third Ave., New York, NY 10017, 800-344-4867, www.nationalmssociety.org.

National Organization for Rare Disorders, Inc. (NORD), P.O. Box 8923, New Fairfield, CT 06812-8923, 203-746-6518, www.rarediseases.org. Search "Rare Diseases Database—Alphabetical Listing;" scroll down to Corticobasal, Pick's disease, etc., for brief information about the disease and information about organizations offering help. There is a small charge for full-text reports.

National Parkinson Foundation, Bob Hope Parkinson Research Center, 1501 N.W. 9th Ave., Bob Hope Rd., Miami, FL 33136-1494, 800-327-4545, www.parkinson.org.

NINDS (National Institute of Neurological Disorders and Stroke), National Institutes of Health, 31 Center Dr., Bethesda, MD 20892, www.ninds.nih.gov. Fact sheets on Pick's disease, dementia with Lewy bodies, progressive supranuclear palsy, corticobasal degeneration.

Society for Progressive Supranuclear Palsy, Woodholme Medical Bldg., suite 515, 1828 Greene Tree Rd., Baltimore, MD 21208, 410-486-3330; 800-457-4777, Canada toll-free: 866-457-4777, www.psp.org.

We Move, 204 West 84th St., New York, NY 10024, 800-437-MOV2, www.wemove.org. A comprehensive resource for movement disorder information and the hub of movement disorder.

NURSING HOME AND ASSISTED LIVING

CMS, formerly the Health Care Financing Administration/HCFA, is the federal agency that oversees all nursing home care and Medicare and Medicaid funding. www.cms.hhs.gov.

Centers for Medicare and Medicaid Services, 7500 Security Blvd., Baltimore, MD 21244-1850, toll free number 877-267-2323.

Consumer Consortium on Assisted Living, 2342 Oak St., Falls Church, VA 22046, 703-533-8121, www.ccal.org.

National Citizens Coalition for Nursing Home Reform. 1424 16th St., N.W., Ste. 202, Washington, DC 20036, 202-332-2275, www.nccnhr.org.

SPEECH AND HEARING

ASHA: American Speech and Hearing Association, 10801 Rockville Pike, Rockville, MD 20852, 800-498-2071, www.asha.org

WEB SITES

Alzheimer's Research Forum, www.alzforum.org. Founded in 1996 to create on-line scientific community dedicated to developing treatments and preventions for Alzheimer's disease

Emedicine, www.emedicine.com. See Anna M. Barrett, M.D., "Pick's Disease," *eMedicin Journal* 2, no. 11 (Nov. 27, 2001).

PubMed, a service of the National Library of Medicine, National Institutes of

Health, provides access to MEDLINE citations and includes links to many sites providing full-text articles and other related resources, www.ncbi.nlm.nih.gov. Click on "PubMed"; search on PubMed for Pick's disease, frontotemporal dementia, Lewy body, etc.

Suggested Reading

GENERAL READING

Books

Doernberg, M. *Stolen Mind: The Slow Disappearance of Ray Doernberg.* Chapel Hill, N.C.: Algonquin Books, 1989. A personal story.

Erb, C. A. *Losing Lou-Ann.* Brandon, Vt.: Holistic Education Press, 1996. A personal story.

Mace, N., and P. Rabins. *The 36-Hour Day*, rev. ed. Baltimore: Johns Hopkins University Press, 1991.

MEDICAL FOCUS

Books

Beinfield, H., and E. Korngold. *Between Heaven and Earth: A Guide to Chinese Medicine.* New York: Ballantine, 1992.

Kaptchuk, T. *The Web That Has No Weaver: Understanding Chinese Medicine,* 2d ed. Lincolnwood, Ill.: Contemporary Books, 2000.

Kertesz , A., and D. G. Munoz, eds. *Pick's Disease and Pick Complex.* Chichester, U.K.: Wiley-Liss, 1998.

Articles

Chow, Tiffany. "How to recognize frontotemporal dementia." *Neuropsychiatry Reviews* 3, no. 3 (April 2002). Tiffany Chow, M.D., a member of the Work Group on Frontotemporal Dementia and Pick's Disease, describes key manifestations of FTD and suggests tips that can aid diagnosis. She also offers advice on how to treat the behavioral and cognitive components of FTD. The article can be found on the Web at www.neuropsychiatryreviews.com/apr02/recognzie.html.

Connections 9, no. 4 (March 2002). *Connections* is published by ADEAR (Alzheimer's Disease Education and Research), National Institute on Aging, P.O. Box 8250, Silver Spring, MD 20907-8250, 800-438-4380. This issue of *Connections*, dedicated to frontotemporal dementia, is online at www.alzheimers.org/pubs/conv09n4.html.

Grossman, Murray. "A Multidisciplinary approach to Pick's disease and frontotemporal dementia." *Neurology* 56, no. 11, suppl. 4 (2001).

McKhann, Guy M., et al. "Clinical and pathological diagnosis of frontotemporal dementia: Report of the work group on frontotemporal dementia and Pick's disease." *Archives of Neurology* 58, no. 11 (Nov. 2001).

"Once confused with Alzheimer's, frontotemporal dementia strikes patients earlier, causing changes in communication, cognition, and personality." *John Douglas French Center Journal* 10: 2–5. This article is available through the Pick's Disease Support Group (CANDID) Web site at www.pdsg.org.uk/articles/JDFC-1.htm.

Snowden, Julie S., David Neary, and David M. A. Mann. "Frontotemporal dementia." *British Journal of Psychiatry* 180 (2002). This overview of clinical and pathological characteristics of frontotemporal dementia and its nosological status can be downloaded at www.psychiatry.wustl.edu/Resources/LiteratureList/ 2002/February/Snowden.pdf.

MANAGING DAILY CARE

Books

Alzheimer's Association. *Activity Programming for Persons with Dementia: A Sourcebook*. Chicago: Alzheimer's Association, 1995.

Dunn, H. *Hard Choices for Loving People: CPR, Artificial Feeding, Comfort Measures Only, and the Elderly Patient*, 3d ed. Herendon, Va.: A and A Publisher, 1994.

Robinson, A., B. Spencer, and L. White. *Understanding Difficult Behaviors: Some Practical Suggestions for Coping with Alzheimer's Disease and Related Disorders.* Ypsilanti, Mich.: Michigan State University, 1988. Check with your local Alzheimer's Association chapter for availability.

Martin, J., and J. Backhouse. *Goodlooking, Easy Swallowing Cookbook.* Woburn, Mass.: Butterworth-Heinemann, 1993.

Perrin, T., and H. May. *Well-being in Dementia: An Occupational Approach for Therapists and Careers.* Edinburgh, U.K.: Churchill Livingstone, 2000.

Wilson, R. J. *Non-chew Cookbook.* Minneapolis: Wilson Publishing, 1985.

Zgola, J. M. *Doing Things: A Guide to Programming Activities for Persons with Alzheimer's Disease and Related Disorders.* Baltimore: Johns Hopkins University Press, 1987.

CAREGIVER RESOURCES

Book

Cohen, Marion., *Dear Aunt S: How to Ask for Help from Family and Friends in Time of Crisis.* Brooklyn, N.Y.: Center for Thanatology Research, 2003.

CARING FOR YOURSELF

Books

Kushner, H. S. *When Bad Things Happen to Good People.* New York: Schocken, 1981.

Lewis, C. S. *A Grief Observed.* New York: Harper and Row, 1963.

Index

causes of, 37, 38, 50
corticobasal degeneration (CBD), 33, 41, 46–47, 57, 119, 206
Creutzfeldt-Jakob disease (CJD), 37, 134

deconditioning, 95
  cardiovascular and pulmonary problems, 96–97
  contractures, 95
  loss of muscle strength and endurance, 95
  pressure sores, 96
  prevention and treatments, 109–110
dementia. *See also* frontotemporal dementia
  causes of, 32, 36, 37–38
  definition of, 29–32
  diagnosing, 38–39
  drug-induced, 38, 53
  early diagnosis of, 32, 37
  with Lewy bodies (DLB), 34, 37, 38, 134
  presenile, 31, 35 (*see also* senile)
  semantic, 33, 42–43, 47, 78, 80
  testing for, 38 (*see also* imaging)
    electroencephalogram (EEG), 38, 50, 70
depression
  versus apathy, 212
  in caregivers, 306, 309
  and cognitive slowness, 38, 53
  pharmacologic therapy for, 51, 78, 79, 86, 141, 227
  and psychotherapy, 84
  and social isolation, 169, 170
DNA
  APP gene, 131
  and chromosomes, 58, 59
  and genes, 58
    autosomal dominant conditions, 59, 61

autosomal recessive conditions, 59–60
MAPT gene, 61–62, 63, 132 (*see also* tau protein)
mutations, 39, 59, 64, 132
  and genotype/phenotype correlations, 62
polymorphisms, 59
  haplotypes, 62
durable medical equipment (DME), 103–106, 113

elderly, 34, 38, 40, 121
environmental modifications, 193–202

family medical history, 56–57
Food and Drug Administration (FDA), 76, 85, 86
  Center for Drug Evaluation and Research, 85
frontotemporal dementia (FTD). *See also* dementia
  and behavioral interventions, 51, 83–84, 99, 121
  causes of, 41, 52, 55
  and causes of death, 48, 121
  clinical criteria for, 52–53
  comparison to Alzheimer's disease, 40
  definition of, 32–33
  and disorders of affect and social comportment, 44–45, 47, 52
  disorders that mimic, 50–51
  early onset of, 49, 52, 61, 122
  and environmental triggers, 140
  and ethics, 221–22, 235, 240
  family history of, 61, 64, 142
  features of, 40, 41–42, 47–48, 52–53, 101–102, 119–20, 162, 182
    hallucinations, 34, 40, 51
    incontinence, 48, 96, 255